Prof. Arnold Ehret's

RATIONAL FASTING
FOR PHYSICAL, MENTAL, AND
SPIRITUAL REJUVENATION:

Introduced & Edited by Prof. Spira

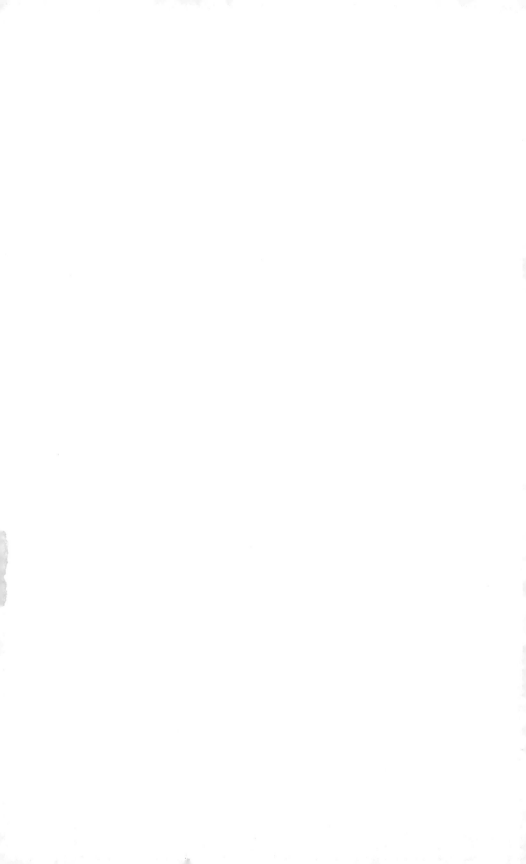

PROF. ARNOLD EHRET'S RATIONAL FASTING FOR PHYSICAL, MENTAL, AND SPIRITUAL REJUVENATION: INTRODUCED AND EDITED BY PROF. SPIRA

By Prof. Arnold Ehret

Introduced and Edited by Prof. Spira

With Articles by Fred S. Hirsch and Teresa Mitchell

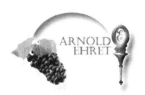

Published by Breathair Publishing 2014

Columbus, Ohio

First Edition

General Disclaimer: The content found in this document and related websites is based upon the opinions and research of the authors and is strictly for informational and educational purposes only. If you choose to use the material in this book on yourself, the authors and publishers take no responsibility for your actions and decisions or the consequences thereof. The content is not intended to replace a one-on-one relationship with a qualified health care professional and is not intended as medical advice. It is intended as a sharing of knowledge, information about health, and opinions based on the research and experiences of the authors and their collaborators.

Breathair Publishing
Columbus, Ohio

Available from www.mucusfreelife.com, Amazon.com, Kindle, and other retail outlets

Printed in the United States of America

First Edition, 2014

ISBN-13: 978-0-99-065642-5
ISBN-10: 0-99-065642-X

www.mucusfreelife.com

Contents

Introduction by Prof. Spira

Fasting is the omnipotent healing modality for animal life. It is a natural and (should be) an instinctual part of life. Yet, nothing is mired in more controversy, misinformation, and miseducation than the subject of fasting. Today, there is little consensus among natural health seekers and practitioners as to what truly constitutes fasting. For some, a diet of mucus-free fruits and vegetables (the mucusless diet) may be considered a level of fasting. For others, a liquid diet of fruit and vegetable juices is a fast. Some assert that consuming only water is true fasting. Yet, others say that dry fasting (no liquids or solid food) is the only real way to fast.

We need not look any further than the works of Prof. Arnold Ehret to find a rational and practical approach to understand what fasting is and how to do it. Ehret does not have a strict or dogmatic definition of what fasting is and is not. In this book, as well its companion text *Mucusless Diet Healing System*, Ehret discusses a spectrum of fasting experiences, including water, juice, and all-fruit dieting. As a general definition, Ehret asserts that fasting is "simply eating less."

The word "fast" means to abstain from or restrict the intake of drink and/or food for a period of time. It may also refer to various forms of dietary restriction, which include abstaining from solid foods (juice or liquid fasting), mucus-forming foods (mucusless diet), animal products, and so forth. Fasting is a dynamic concept and may

1

also refer more broadly to abstaining from modern conveniences or unnatural additions, for example, a fast from electricity or the use of electronics for a period of time. In addition to health and healing purposes, various forms of fasting have been a part of many spiritual and religious traditions. Christianity, Judaism, Jainism, Buddhism, Hinduism, Taoism, Islam, Ancient Egyptian Mystery Schools, and more all have strong fasting traditions and many propagate various forms or degrees of fruit dieting.

From Ehret's perspective, fasting for humans in our current pathological conditions is a relative proposition. Ultimately, it is important to understand the various levels of fasting available to you. What fasting is for one person's body may not be the same for someone else. As Ehret implied, for some, just eating a mucusless or a fruit-only diet could be a level of fasting. And what is and is not fasting to a person's body may shift over time as a person's physiology changes. To determine which fasting regimen is right for you, it is essential to understand the content within this book, which remains the quintessential book on the subject. Through dedicated study and practice you will learn to fast safely and effectively in order to overcome and prevent a myriad of physical and mental illnesses.

Fasting as an Art Form

Fasting may be viewed as a grand art form. There is much more to fasting than merely going without food or drink. Learning to begin a fast properly is very important. Transitioning from a poor to an improved diet before initiating a fast can allow the process to be much more effective. Understanding the role of colon irrigation (enemas) in relationship to fasting is vital. As you begin, it is important to consider the following questions: What is the amount of uneliminated waste in your bowels? Do you have a uric-acid/lean body type or a fatty/mucus body type? (See the *Mucusless Diet Healing System* for more on body types.) What is the nature of the uneliminated fecal matter still encased in your bowels? Is it made up of the residue of pus-forming foods such as meat and dairy products? Or, are your internal impurities the residue of plant-based, mucus-free foods such as fat- and starch-free fruits and vegetables? Answers to these questions will help you intuitively make rational decisions before, during, and after the fasting process.

2

There is no greater task within the fasting arts than the ability to eloquently break one's fast. Fasting too long for your physiological condition only to uncontrollably break it with mucus-forming foods is futile and defeats the purpose of your fast. This is one reason Ehret emphasized "gradual change" toward cleansing mucus-free foods, combined with a series of short, intermittent fasts, for newcomers to fasting and the mucusless diet. As you gain experience with short-term fasting, you will learn how to maintain total control whenever you begin or break a fast of any length.

Do not feel as if you need to do long dry, water, or juice fasts if you are not physically or mentally ready. Strive to do rational fasts based on the needs of your own body. You need not prove anything to anyone, and fasting is not a competition to see who can be food-free for the longest period of time. A lot of people play basketball, but few people think that they should be able to play like Michael Jordan without serious practice and long-term dedication. Many people play music, but few expect to have the virtuosity of a jazz or concert pianist in a matter of weeks. It takes years of dedicated practice to attain the highest levels of any art form. Yet in dietetics, health seekers often feel as if they should be able to skip over the transitional process and sustain long fasts without dedicated practice. Long-term fasting may be a worthy goal, but it should be achieved through fervent practice over a long time. As Ehret pointed out, most people are far too obstructed with mucus, pus, and toxemias for long-term fasts to be very beneficial.

Concepts and approaches similar to that of a 21-day cleanse are problematic and should be avoided. Many people pursue such "cleanses," looking for a quick fix for losing weight or overcoming a particular ailment. Yet, as Ehret says, ill health issues will continue to emerge as long as a person continues to eat poorly after a fast. In this book, Ehret offers the most rational approach to fasting that can easily be adopted as a regular part of life. When fasting and mucusless diet are applied properly, you can permanently transform what foods you desire. Instead of relying on willpower to avoid wrong foods, you will begin to crave more of the right foods.

3

History of Rational Fasting

The earliest English version of this book was entitled *Rational Fasting and Regeneration Diet,* translated from German in 1913. At that time, it was a small book or pamphlet that made up the first part of this edition. In 1922, *Rational Fasting: Regeneration Diet and Natural Cure for All Diseases* was published. By 1926, *Rational Fasting for Physical, Mental, and Spiritual Rejuvenation was* a little over 60 pages and divided into two parts, which are represented under Section I in this edition.

Fred Hirsch, Arnold Ehret's most loyal student and proprietor of Ehret Publishing Company until the 1970s, released subsequent versions—most notably, *Rational Fasting for Physical, Mental, and Spiritual Rejuvenation,* which included one of his own essays, entitled "Health and Happiness through Fasting." Subsequent editions have bundled various articles with *Rational Fasting,* especially "Your Road to Regeneration" by Prof. Arnold Ehret, as well as "My Road to Health" and "Build your own Road to Health" by Teresa Mitchell, both of which are included in this edition.

The Best Way to Use this Book

Rational Fasting goes hand-in-hand with the *Mucusless Diet Healing System.* You are strongly encouraged to read both texts, subsequently. Understanding and practicing the mechanics of the "Transition Diet" found in the *Mucusless Diet Healing System* is of the utmost importance to having the greatest success with Ehret's approach to fasting. I highly recommend examining both books before experimenting with fasting. With that said, this book can and should be read and reread multiple times. The simple yet potent message found in *Rational Fasting* has the power to elevate your consciousness. And for serious practitioners of Ehret's methods, this book will seem to transform every time you read it. Of course, it is you—not the book—that is transforming. As you transform your body and mind through fasting and mucusless diet, you will continually breathe new life into this text. Subtle elements that you may overlook the first time you read the book will come to life as you experience improved levels of health and vitality.

The principles found in *Rational Fasting* are needed today more than ever. In a world where natural healing methods have been largely forsaken by the masses, Ehret sheds light on the powerful art of fasting and its supreme role in regenerating the human body, mind, and spirit.

-Prof. Spira

Summer 2014

Preface

Are you one of the thousands of present-age persons discouraged and disheartened because of ill health? Is your faith in so-called cures shattered after having tried them without results? Are you only able to use a small percentage of the vitality that good Mother Nature endows her beloved ones with? Probably you have been told that only an operation will save you. Somehow, when we suffer organic trouble, we fail to think clearly and permit ourselves to be easily persuaded into operations. If you are one of these unfortunates, DON'T GIVE UP HOPE. For "he or she that hath health hath hope, and he or she that hath hope, hath everything."

"Since humans degenerated through civilization, they no longer know what to do when they become sick." The genuine principles of healing are simple and few. Our very lack of appetite, which occurs when we are sick, is Nature's method of teaching her children. One might properly call this a "forced fast." These are but a few of the truisms taught by Arnold Ehret in his many writings. Our greatest possession is health.

A general agreement seems to be gaining acceptance among an increasing number of practitioners both of the drugless, as well as the medical, fraternity that the fundamental cause of disease is the presence of foreign material in the human body, but it has not as yet led to the discovery of the roots of this invading mystery. Prof. Ehret has conclusively proven that this disease-causing material is the undigested, uneliminated, and decayed, rotting food elements resulting from too much eating of wrong foods. It is therefore entirely reasonable and should be clearly seen that the main factor in the health enigma should consist of dietetics. If overeating is the main cause of the patient's disease, it requires intelligently conducted fasts to correct the condition. It is a known fact that all of the animal kingdom living in a natural environment instinctively heal themselves through fasting. It can be easily proven that a person living on a mixed diet of animal flesh and starchy vegetables has a system more or less clogged with mucus. This condition has been going on since early childhood—in fact, even before. These foods are not suitable for humankind, and they form a sticky, gluey consistency that eventually clogs the circulation. Is it not self-evident and certainly reasonable that this disease-producing eating must be stopped! Fasting, plus a decrease in the quantity of food eaten daily, is the only check on overeating. Exercise due precaution not to proceed too rapidly, for an unwise application of the eliminative process could cause a serious condition to develop.

This drugless healing is not limited in its scope; and through its proper application and use, it restores normal functioning, overcoming practically all ailments to which the human family is subject.

"TRUTH WEARS NO MASK. BOWS AT NO HUMAN SHRINE, SEEKS NEITHER PLACE NOR APPLAUSE; SHE ASKS ONLY A HEARING." —*Redfield*

—Fred S. Hirsch

SECTION I

RATIONAL Fasting

By Prof. Arnold Ehret

Part I

The Common Fundamental Cause
in the Nature of Diseases

All the phases of the process of development of medical science, including those of the earliest periods of civilization, have in their way of understanding the causal nature of diseases, that one thing in common: i.e., that the diseases, owing to external causes, enter into the human body and thus, by force of a necessary or at least unavoidable law, disturb the body in its existence, cause it pain and at last destroy it. Even modern medical science, no matter how scientifically enlightened it pretends to be, has not quite turned away from this basic note of demonic interpretation. In fact, the most modern achievement, bacteriology, rejoices over every newly discovered bacillus as a further addition to the army of beings whose accepted task it is to endanger the life of humans.

Looking at it from a philosophical standpoint, this interpretation differs from the medieval superstition and the period of fetishism only in the supplemental name. Formerly it was an "evil spirit," which

9

imagination went so far as to believe in "satanic personages"; now this same dangerous monster is a microscopically visible being whose existence has been proven beyond any doubt.

The matter, it is true, has still a great drawback in the so-called "disposition"—a fine word! But what we really are to understand by it, nobody has ever told us. All the tests on animals, with their symptom-reactions, do not prove anything sure, because these occur only by means of injection into the blood circulation, and never by introduction into the digestive channel through the mouth.

There is something true in the conception of "external invasion" of a disease, as well as in heredity; however, not in the sense that the invader is a spirit (demon) hostile to life, or a microscopic being (bacillus), but all *diseases* without exception, even the hereditary, are caused—disregarding a few other hygienic causes—by biologically wrong, "unnatural" food, and by each ounce of overnourishment, only and exclusively.

First of all, I maintain that in all diseases without exception there exists a tendency by the organism to secrete mucus, and in case of a more advanced stage—pus (decomposed blood). Of course, every healthy organism must also contain a certain mucus—lymph, a fatty substance of the bowels, etc., of a mucus nature. Every expert will admit this in all catarrhalic cases, from a harmless cold in the nose to inflammation of the lungs and consumption,[1] as well as in epilepsy (attacks showing froth at the mouth, mucus). Where this secretion of mucus does not show freely and openly, as in cases of ear, eye, skin or stomach trouble; heart diseases; rheumatism; gout; etc., even in all degrees of insanity, mucus is the main factor of the illness. The natural secretive organs unable to cope with it longer, the mucus enters the blood causing heat, inflammation, pain, and fever at the respective spot where the vessel-system is probably contracted owing to an overcooling fever (cold), heat, inflammation, pain, fever, etc.

---

[1] "Consumption" is an archaic term for what is currently referred to as pulmonary tuberculosis. Ehret's discussion may also be generally applied to all "obstructive lung diseases," which are respiratory illness characterized by airway obstruction. Terms used to denote various forms of constipation of the lungs include asthma, bronchiectasis, bronchitis, and chronic obstructive pulmonary disease (COPD).

We need only to give a patient of any kind nothing but "mucusless" food, for instance, fruit or even nothing but water or lemonade. We then find that the entire digestive energy, freed for the first time, throws itself upon the mucus-matters, accumulated since childhood and frequently hardened, as well as on the "pathologic beds" formed therefrom. And the result? With unconditional certainty, this mucus, which I mark as the common basic and main cause of all diseases, will appear in the urine and in the excrements. If the disease is already somewhat advanced so that in some spot, even in the innermost interior, there have appeared pathologic beds, i.e., decomposed cellular tissues, then pus is also being secreted. As soon as the introduction of mucus by means of "artificial food," fatty meat, bread, potatoes, farinaceous products, rice, milk, etc. ceases, the blood circulation attacks the mucus and the pus of the body themselves and secretes them through the urine; and in the case of heavily infected bodies, even through all the openings at their command, as well as through the mucus membranes.

If potatoes, grain-meal, rice, or the respective meat-materials are boiled long enough, we receive jelly-like slime (mucus) or paste used by bookbinders and carpenters. This mucus substance soon becomes sour, ferments, and forms a bed for fungi, molds, and bacilli. In the process of digestion, which is nothing else but a boiling—a combustion—this slime or paste is being secreted in the same manner, for the blood can use only the ex-digested sugar transformed from starch. The secreted matter, the superfluous product, i.e., this paste or slime, is being completely excreted in the beginning. It is, therefore, easy to understand that in the course of life the intestines and the stomach are gradually being pasted and slimed up to such an extent that this paste of floral and this slime of faunal origin turn into fermentation, clog up the blood vessels and finally decompose the stagnated blood. If figs, dates, or grapes are boiled down thick enough we also receive a pap which, however, does not turn to fermentation and never secretes slime, but which is called syrup. Fruit sugar, the most important thing for the blood, is also sticky, it is true, but is being completely used up by the body as the highest form of fuel, and leaves for excretion only traces of cellulose, which, not being sticky, is promptly excreted and does not ferment. Boiled-down

11

sugar, owing to its resistance against fermentation, is even used for the preservation of food.

Each healthy or sick person deposits on the tongue a sticky mucus as soon as he or she fasts or reduces food. This occurs also on the mucus membrane of the stomach, of which the tongue is an exact copy. In the first stool after fasting, this mucus makes its appearance.

I recommend to my reader or to the physicians and searchers to test my claims by way of experiments, which alone are entitled to real scientific recognition. The experiment, the question put to nature, is the basis of a natural science and reveals the infallible truth, no matter whether it is stated by me or somebody else. Furthermore, I recommend the following experiments to those who are brave enough to test on their own bodies, which I undertook on mine. They will receive the same answer from nature, i.e., from their organism, provided that the latter be sound in my sense. "Exact" to a certain degree reacts only to the clean, sound, mucusless organism. After a 2-year strict fruit diet with intercalated fasting cures, I had attained a degree of health which is simply not imaginable nowadays and which allowed of my making the following experiments:

> With a knife, I made an incision in my lower arm. There was no flow of blood as it thickened instantly, closing up the wound; no inflammation, no pain, no mucus and pus: healed up in 3 days, blood crust thrown off. Later, with vegetaric food, including mucus ferments (starch food) but without eggs and milk: the wound bled a little, caused some pain, and pussed slightly; a light inflammation; complete healing only after some time. After that, the same wounding with meat-food and some alcohol: longer bleeding, the blood of a light color, red and thin; inflammation; pain; pussing for several days; and healing only after a 2-day fast.

I have offered myself, of course in vain, to the Prussian Ministry of War for a repetition of this experiment. Why is it that the wounds of the Japanese healed much quicker and better in the Russo-Japanese War than those of the "meat-and-brandy Russians?" Has nobody for 2,000 years ever thought it over why the opening of the artery and even the poison cup could not kill Seneca, after he had despised meat and fasted in prison? It is said that even before that, Seneca fed on nothing but fruit and water.

All disease is finally nothing else but a clogging-up of the smallest blood vessels, the capillaries, by mucus. Nobody will want to clean the water conduit of a city, a pipe system, which is fed with soiled water by a pump, the filters of which are clogged up, without having the water supply shut off during the cleaning process. If the conduit supplies the entire city or a portion of it with unclean water, or if even the smallest branch-pipes are clogged up, there is no human in the world who would repair or improve that respective spot; everybody thinks at once of the central, of the tank, and the filters, and these together with the pumping machine can be cleaned only as long as the water supply is shut off.

"I am the Lord, thy physician"—English and modern: nature alone heals, cleans, "unmucuses" best and infallibly sure, but only if the supply, or at least the mucus supply, is stopped. Each "physiological machine," humans like animals, cleanse themselves immediately, dissolving the mucus in the clogged-up vessels, without stopping short as soon as the supply of compact food at least, is interrupted. Even in the case of the supposedly healthy person, this mucus, as already mentioned, then appears in the urine where it can be seen after cooling off in the proper glass tubes! Whoever denies, ignores, or fights this uniform fact, because perhaps it is not in accord with their teachings or is not sufficiently scientific, is jointly guilty of the impossibility of detection of the principal cause of all diseases.

Therewith, I also uncover the last secret of consumption. Or does anybody believe that this enormous quantity of mucus thrown off by a patient stricken with tuberculosis for years and years emanates only from the lung itself? Just because this patient is then almost forcibly fed on "mucus" (pap, milk, fat meats) the mucus can never cease until the lung itself decays and the "bacilli" make their appearance when death becomes inevitable. The mystery of the bacilli is solved simply thus: The gradual clogging-up of the blood vessels by mucus leads to decomposition, to fermentation of these mucus products and "boiled, dead-food" residues. These decay partially on

13

the living body (pussy abscesses, cancer, tuberculosis, syphilis, lupus, etc.). Now everybody knows that meat, cheese, and all organic matter will again "germinate, put forth bacilli" during the process of decomposition. It is for this reason that these germs appear and are detectable only in the more advanced stage of the disease, when, however, they are not the cause but the product of the disease, and disease-furthering only in so far as the decomposition, for instance of the lung, is being hastened by them, because the excretions of the bacilli, their toxins, act poisoning. If it be correct that bacilli invade, "infect" from the exterior, then it is nothing but the mucus that makes possible their activity, and furnishes the proper soil, the "disposition."

As already stated, I have repeatedly (once for 2 years) lived mucusless, i.e., on fruit exclusively. I was no longer in need of a handkerchief, which product of civilization I hardly need even up to this date. Has anyone ever seen a healthy animal living in freedom expectorate or blow its nose? A chronic inflammation of the kidneys, considered deadly, which I was stricken with, was not only healed, but I am enjoying a degree of health and efficiency that by far surpasses even that of my healthiest youth. I want to see the person who, being sick unto death at 31, can run for 2 hours and a quarter without a stop or make an endurance march of 56 hours' duration—8 years later.

It is surely theoretically correct that humans were mere fruit eaters in times gone by, and biologically correct that they can be it even today. Or can the horse sense of humans not conceive without any direct proofs of the fact that humans, before becoming hunters, lived on fruits only? I even maintain that humans lived in absolute health, beauty, and strength without pain and grief, just the way the Bible says. Fruit only, the sole "mucusless" food, is natural. Everything prepared by humans, or supposedly improved by them, are evil. The arguments regarding fruit are scientifically exact; in the apple or banana, for instance, everything can be found contained what humans need. Humans are so perfect that they can live on one kind of fruit only, at least for quite some time. This has been conclusively proven by the mono-diet system of August Engelhardt who solved by his great philosophy and practice of natural life all problems of humankind. But a self-evident truth preached by nature

14

must not be discarded just because no one has been able to apply it in actual practice on account of civilizational considerations. From the eating of fruit only, one gets first a crisis, i.e., cleansing. No human would have ever believed me that it is possible to live without food for 126 days, in which 49 were undertaken at a stretch, during a period covering 14 months. Now I have done it, and yet this truth is not being understood. Hitherto I state and will teach only this fact, that fruit is the most natural "healing remedy." Whether my calculation is correct will be proven by the next epidemic. I take, however, this opportunity to uncover the reasons why the self-evident is not believed in. When in the previous century someone talked about the possibility of phoning from London to Paris, everybody laughed because there had never been such a thing. Natural food is not being believed in anymore, because almost no one practices it and living in today's civilization, we cannot easily practice it. It must also be considered that contra-interests fear that the prices of other, artificial foodstuffs may drop, and others fear that the food physiology may receive a shock and physicians become unnecessary. But, it is just this fasting and fruit cure, which requires very strict observation and instruction—therefore, more doctors and less patients who, however, will gladly pay more if they get well. Thus, the social question regarding doctors is solved—an assertion already made by me publicly in Zurich several years ago.

Almost all fasting attempts fail through ignorance of the fact that with the beginning of the mucusless diet, the old mucus is being excreted so much more forcibly until that person is absolutely clean and healthy. THUS, THE SEEMINGLY HEALTHIEST PERSON HAS FIRST TO PASS THROUGH A CONDITION OF SICKNESS (CLEANSING) or go through an intermediate stage of illness to a higher level of health.

This is the "great-cliff" around which so few vegetarians have failed to go—discarding the basic truth just like the mass of people are doing. I have proven this fact in the "Vegetarische Warte," completely on the basis of experiments and facts; and refuting their greatest objection, that of undernourishment, by an actual fasting experiment of 49 days with a preceding fruit diet. My state of health was greatly improved through this radical excretion of mucus, disregarding a few unhygienic circumstances during the test. I

15

received numerous letters of appreciation, especially from the educated classes. The mass of adherents of vegetarianism "mucuses" gaily ahead. Contrasting herewith, it can only be said that the poisons (so-called by them)—meat, alcohol, coffee, and tobacco—are in the long run comparatively harmless, AS LONG AS THEY ARE USED MODERATELY.

In order to avoid misunderstanding on the part of teetotalers and vegetarians, I must insert here a few explanations. Meat is not a foodstuff but only a stimulant that ferments, decays in the stomach. The process of decay, however, does not begin in the stomach, but at once after the slaughtering. This has already been proven on living persons by Prof. Dr. S. Graham, and I complete this fact by saying that meat acts as a stimulant just by means of these poisons of decay, and therefore is being erroneously regarded as a strengthening foodstuff. Or is there anyone who can show me chemico-physiologically that the albumen molecule going through the process of decay is being newly reformed in the stomach and celebrates its resurrection in some muscle of the human body? Like alcohol, the meat produces in the beginning stimulating strength and energy until the entire organism is penetrated by it and the breakdown inevitable. All the other stimulants act likewise. This, therefore, is a false delusion.

The fundamental evil of all non-vegetaric forms of diet consist always in the overeating of meat, as it is the origin of all the other evils, especially in the craving for alcohol. If fruit is eaten almost exclusively, the eagerness for cup or glass loses itself to chastise against it, simply because meat produces the demon thirst. Alcohol is a proven kind of antidote for meat, and the gourmand of the big city, who eats practically nothing but meat, must therefore have wines, mocha, and Havana in order to at least in some way counteract the heavy meat poisoning. It is a well-known fact that, after an opulent dinner, one feels decidedly fresher, physically and mentally, if the stimulants, poisonous in themselves, are taken moderately rather than to stuff one's self full with the "good-eating" to the very fatigue.

I ABSOLUTELY DECLARE WAR ON MEAT AND ALCOHOL; through fruit and moderate eating, these great evils are radically diminished. But whoever finds it impossible to entirely give

16

up meat and alcohol is, if he or she takes them moderately, still far ahead of the vegetaric "over or excess eater." The American, Fletcher, proved this most evidently by his tremendous success, and his secret is explained by my experiments, which show that a person becomes most efficient and develops best in health if he or she eats as little as possible! Are not the oldest people as a rule the poorest? Have not the greatest discoverers and inventors sprung from poverty, i.e., been "little eaters"? Were not the greatest of humankind—the prophets, founders of religions, etc.—ascetics? Is that culture to dine excellently thrice a day, and is it social progress that each working man and woman eats five times a day and then pumps themselves full with beer or wine at night? If the sick organism can regenerate by eating nothing, I think the logical consequence is that a healthy organism needs but little food in order to remain healthy, strong, and persevering.

All so-called miracles of the saints have their only origin in ascetics, and are today impossible but for the simple reason that, although much praying is done, no fasting is adhered to. This is the only solution of this quarrel. We have no more miracles because we have no more saints, i.e., sanctified and healed by ascetics and fastings. The saints were self-shining, expressed in modern language: medial or radioactive, but only because through asceticism, they were "godly" healthy, and not "by special grace." I just wish to mention here that I myself have succeeded in visible, electric effluences, but only by external and internal sun energies (sunbaths and food from the "sun kitchen," fruit).

The entire world is quarreling now regarding these questions and miracles. And here is the solution on the basis of experiments, which everybody can repeat if they are brave enough. But it is apparently easier to write books, preach, and pray, or to say that I am an exception. This is true, but only so far as pluck and understanding are concerned. Physiologically, all people are equal, and whoever cannot be moderate may learn it from me if he or she wishes to be a real searcher after health. If a person eats little and is healthy, they can, for quite a length of time, digest the most absurd food, meat, and starch (mucus), i.e., they can again excrete it. Naturally, they become and remain still more perfect and clean if they eat but little fruit, and of this, they need the least because it is the most perfect food. This eternal truth by natural law: humans of today will not and cannot admit, and have a well-founded fear of it, because they are built up of dead-boiled food and their cells die off and are excreted as soon as they sunbathe, fast, or eat the living cells of fruit. But this cure must be done with the greatest care. The duty of medicine is to protect humans from a breakdown of their cells, to hold them above water as long as this is possible only to cause them to die of the disease so much more promptly and quickly, which today is fervently wished for. Vegetarianism cannot deny that the consumers of meat and alcohol can also boast of much health and great deeds and high age, but taken individually and as a people only so long as but little is eaten and no overnourishment caused. Eating "too much" takes less revenge in case of meat eating because meat contains proportionally less "mucus" than starch-containing, "mucus" vegetaric food and the celebrated vegetaric dinners with entirely too many dishes daily. I myself have not cared for many years for any meals; I eat only when I have appetite and then so little that it does not cause any harmful effect, if, on account of an experiment, I am obliged to eat something, which in itself is not entirely free from objection.

If the most serious diseases can be cured by fasting—which has been proven in thousands of cases—and if during the fast one becomes stronger "if it is done right," then the most energetic food, the fruit, should cause one so much the more to become strong and healthy. This has also been scientifically proven by the merited Dr. Bircher. It is true, the science of cure by nature has recognized the fact that something must get out of the sick organism; but it has so far ascribed the greatest importance to physical stimulations, ignoring completely the real natural moment to the process of cure, the abstaining from food, and through following a fruit diet. At least, they have only offered a substitute by a non-alcohol and meatless diet. This does not mean much in the face of my "mucus-theory." And what is this mucusless alcohol not accused of today? It will soon be made the "scapegoat" of all diseases because here and there is found a depraved one who, consuming it in enormous quantities, ends in delirium. Just compel a drinker to fast a few days or to eat nothing but fruit—I will wager that the best glass of beer will have lost its flavor for him or her. This proves that the entire "civilized" mess, from beefsteak down to apparently harmless oatmeal, creates the desire for these detested antidotes: alcohol, coffee, tea, tobacco. Why? Because much-eating paralyzes, and only the use of stimulants restores!

Here is the true and fundamental reason for the increase of alcohol consumption: the overnourishment, especially with meat. Prof. Dr. Graham says in his "Physiology of Nourishment," "A drinker can reach a high age, a glutton never." This is true, because the acute alcohol acts as a stimulant; and especially the modern beer is less harmful in the long run than the chronic stuffing up of the digestive channel with mucus-forming food.

I now ask: what appeals more to reason—to wipe out the masses of mucus, piled up since childhood or having infected the cellular tissues of the body by poisonous drugs or parts cut away by useless, avoidable operations; having the cure delayed by one-sided osteopathy; chiropractic malpractice misunderstood electrical treatments; mucus-forming and often unclean milk cures; weakening hot springs treatments; the Christian Science superstition; etc.; or simply to stop the further supply of mucus caused by unnatural diet? Or is there anybody who would like to prove to me that the most skillful chef or confectioner is capable of producing something better than an apple, a grape, or a banana? If nourishment by mucus and overeating is the true fundamental cause of all diseases without exception, which I can prove to anybody on his or her own body, then there can exist but one natural remedy, i.e., fasting and fruit diet. That every animal fasts in case of even the slightest uneasiness, is a well-known fact. And to culture, and thanks to humans feeding them, domestic animals have lost their sharp instinct for the right kind of food and the natural hours of feeding—and therewith their proper state of health and acuteness of sense—they will nevertheless when sick, accept only the most necessary food; they fast themselves back to health. Poor, sick people, however, must under no circumstances live on short rations for more than 1 or 2 days, for fear that they may "lose strength."

Already many leading physicians have called fasting wonder cures, cure of the uncured, cure of all cures, etc. Certain charlatans have brought this infallible, but at the same time dangerous, cure to discredit. I have done in fasting the most significant thing in centuries: 49 days, world-record (see "Vegetarische Warte," 1909, Books 19, 20, 22; 1920, Books 1 and 2). Furthermore, I am the only one who combines this cure with systematically and individually adapted fruit diet, which makes it astonishingly easier and absolutely harmless. We are, therefore, undoubtedly put in a position to heal diseases that the school of medicine designates as incurable. On the basis of my deduction that this mucus coming from cultured food is the fundamental cause and main factor in the nature of all diseases, symptoms of age, obesity, falling out of the hair, wrinkles, weakness of nerves and memory, etc., there is justified hope for the creation of a new phase of development of the progressive healing methods and biological medicine.

Already Hippocrates had uniformly recognized the "disease material" for all diseases. Prof. Jaeger has defined the "common" as "stench," but had not discovered the source of this "bad smell." Dr. Lahmann and other representatives of the physical dietetic tendency, especially Kuhne, came on to the tracks of the "common foreign matter." But not one of them showed, recognized, or proved by experiment that it is this very mucus of culture food that loads up our organism from childhood and attacks it at a certain degree of fermentation, forms pathologic beds, i.e., decomposes the cellular tissue of the body itself into pus and decay. It is being mobilized in case of casual colds or high temperatures, etc., and produces, in its tendency to leave the body, symptoms of abnormal functions, which hitherto have been regarded as the disease itself. It is, therefore, for the first time possible to define what is meant by "decomposition." The more the "mucus" (bad mother's milk and all its substitutes) is being administered from childhood on, or the less this mucus is being excreted owing to hereditary weakness through the organs made to perform this task, the greater is the inclination to catch cold, fever, to freeze, to admit parasites, to get sick, and to prematurely grow old. Very likely, by this the veil has been lifted from the secret, which hitherto has always surrounded the nature of the white corpuscles. I believe that here, as in many other cases, we are confronted with an error of medical science. The bacteria throw themselves upon the white corpuscles, composed to the largest extent of this mucus denounced by me. Are not the bacteria being bred on this mucus by the millions outside of the organism?—on potatoes, broth, gelatin, i.e., on mucus, i.e., nitrogenous, vegetable or animal substances consisting of an alkalically-reacting fluid containing granulated cells of the appearance of the white blood-corpuscles? Perhaps in an entirely healthy condition the so-called mucus membrane should not at all be white, slimy, but clean and red like on animals. Perhaps this "corpse mucus" is even the cause of the paleness of the white race! Paleface! Corpse color!

With this "mucus theory" to be confirmed by experiment, the specter "disease" has been finally deprived of its demonic mask. The persons who believe me can heal not only themselves if everything else fails, but we have for the first time been given the means to radically prevent disease and to make it definitely impossible. Even the dream of lasting youth and beauty is now about to become true.

The animal, and especially the human organism, is, from a mechanical standpoint, a complicated tube system of blood vessels with air-gas impetus by means of the lungs, in which the blood fluid is constantly kept moving and regulated by the heart as a valve. The decomposition of the air-gas is accomplished by each breath in the lungs (separating of the air into oxygen and nitrogen); thus, the blood is constantly kept moving and the human body does its service incredibly long without fatigue. Let nobody come to me with the silly excuse of the "daily experience of the absolutely natural compulsion of much-eating," prescribed for working people, etc., before it has not been experienced by such complainant how long it is possible to work or march, without fatigue, after fasting or fruit food. Fatigue is, in the first place, a reducing of strength by too much digestion work; secondly, a clogging-up of the heated and consequently narrowed-down blood vessels; and thirdly, a "self-and re-poisoning" through the excretion of mucus during the motion. All organic substances of animal origin excrete cyanate groups in their decomposition, which the chemist Hensel has defined as bacilli proper. The air is not only the highest and most perfect operating material of the human body, but simultaneously the first element for the erection, repair, substitute, and very likely, the animal organism derives nitrogen also from the air. On certain caterpillars, an increase of weight through air alone has been stated.

Complete fasting, followed by a decrease in the quantity of food eaten, is the only check on "overeating." And a diet of "non-mucus-forming" foods must replace the "mucus-forming" foods. Fresh, tree-ripened fruits and the green-leaf starchless vegetables have been long recognized and my *Mucusless Diet Healing System* is already a well-proven fact! Neither fasting nor the fruit diet has been accepted by the medical authorities, nor have they been used by others in strict accordance with the condition of the patient; yet when properly combined as a "systematic cleansing," the treatment has been remarkably successful and satisfactory. The degree of the individual's weakness, together with the disturbing sensations experienced by the patient, is an extremely important factor that must be given full consideration. My cure is the only one on record that can be regulated and controlled as to speed!

Remedies for the Removal of the Common Fundamental Cause of
Diseases and the Prevention of Their Re-occurrence

After having told my readers the dread and horror of being sick or getting sick in the previous chapter, it befits me to show them the means and ways, as far as this, commonly speaking, is possible, how to successfully encounter mucus-poisoning, this greatest foe of health. Here I wish to show three means and ways that can produce a beneficial change.

1. The shortest and best way is the fasting so much talked about in this book. It cuts short the life of the "grim misdoer" in our body and causes him to flee, and he leaves us faster with fright and terror.

Healthy people can submit themselves to a fasting cure without any further ceremony. It goes without saying that they must fast reasonably and assume personal responsibility, and not cause dangerous overexertions during the fasting period by demanding of themselves physical or mental performances that they could not live up to even at full fare. I insert here a precautionary measure which must be observed in all fasting cures: the complete emptying of the bowels at the beginning of the fasting by harmless purgative (such as an aromatic herb compound), or by a syringe, or by both. It lies in the nature of the thing that the person who fasts must not be bothered by gas or decomposing matter that form from the excrements remaining in the bowels; it suffices that the mucus during the excretion gives him enough trouble, as already stated.

If it is not desired to take a more prolonged fast, although he or she is healthy, one should try a short one. Even a fasting of 36 hours one or two times weekly can be depended upon to produce very favorable results. It is best to start by leaving off the supper and taking an enema instead.

Then, in the case of a 36-hour fast, nothing is eaten until the following morning, the meal to consist of nothing but fruits. The eating of fruit is desirable after each fasting, as the juices of the fruits cause a moving of the mucus masses, which have loosened. However, let me caution all, especially the sick and elderly people: this treatment must be carefully individualized.

One arrives at this result much sooner, however, if a longer fasting is done in the way described, for instance, 3 days, and then continues what I call an after-fasting cure. That is, do not eat anything for 3 days and drink only fresh lemonade, unsugared, in single gulps as may become necessary, and begin on the fourth day with some fruits. At the close of the fourth day, take a thorough enema. More fruit may be added from day to day, until about the seventh day of the "after-cure" the normal quantity of fruit diet in the proper composition and selection has been reached. The fasting, however, can be extended for weeks by healthy persons and by those whose occupation permits of their spending their time in bed in case of difficult excretions of mucus. Nobody should seriously object to the so-called "bad looks" or the decrease in weight. The body fasts itself into health, despite the miserable complexion, and in a remarkably short time the cheeks will be adorned by a healthy, natural red. The weight is also restored to its normal standard very soon after the fasting. After a fast, the body reacts on every ounce of food. Very moderate eaters and frequently fasting people have a very fine, spiritual expression of the face. It is said that Pope Leo XIII, that great faster and life-artist, had a very clear, almost transparent complexion.

In this connection, I wish to call attention to another point already mentioned elsewhere, for the success of the fasting depends upon it to a great extent. The fasting person must not unnecessarily become depressed or ill humored; the one condition finds relief in the disagreeable moments by complete rest, the other by quick and decided work, especially in light and mechanical occupation.

When the body has been ridden of the mucus, slime, and paste, then it is the sacred duty of the person who has regained health to keep up the reclaimed highest earthly happiness and to guard it by means of natural, correct food. On this subject, a few short remarks in the following paragraphs will not come amiss.

2. The person who cannot fast because of considerations of advanced lung or heart trouble, for instance, may at least see to it that the further accumulation of mucus be cut short by refraining from pronounced mucus-formers, especially from all flour (cake), rice, potato dishes, boiled milk, cheese, meat, etc. Whoever cannot miss bread entirely must eat black or white bread only toasted; by toasting, the bread loses much of its harmfulness, as the mucus substances are partly destroyed. The eating of toasted bread or whole-wheat Zwieback has the further advantage that not much can be eaten of it; it cannot be devoured as wild beasts do, and the necessary chewing will fatigue even the greediest gums. Whoever cannot bite the toasted bread on account of bad teeth may suck on it until it dissolves—a splendid way to restore declined strength. Whoever cannot miss potatoes should eat them only baked, and be sure to eat the jackets.

What then remains for "nutritious food" after I am to give up all albuminous food, like dried peas, lentils, beans, as much as possible? Thus, many a reader will ask with a sigh.

As to the value of meat, I have set forth my views elsewhere. The slight requirements in albumen are fully covered by sugary fruits; the banana, the nuts, combined with a few figs or dates are first class muscle-formers and strength-givers.

The vegetable (cut small and made into salad), the salads themselves, prepared with oil and plenty of fresh lemon juice, and all the splendid fruits and berries, including those of the South, are worthy of being served on the tables of Gods. And when springtime comes and last season's fruits, especially apples, are on the decline and the new vegetables not yet ready, does not Mother Nature help us out abundantly with oranges from the South? Will the aroma and wealth of these splendid products of nature not induce humans to eventually become a fruit eater entirely?

It is not possible for me to go into the question of food and its effects exhaustively in this book; for healthy people these statements may suffice; to sick people I recommend special prescriptions according to their state of health. If you are not already an owner of my *Mucusless Diet Healing System* Lesson Course, may I suggest that you secure a copy of this book. It may be mentioned that non-fasters and people easily succumbing to illness may at least follow the morning fastings or non-breakfast plan. It would be better for all concerned not to eat anything before 10:00 a.m. and then nothing but fruits. The reward for this little self-chastising will certainly show itself shortly—especially if the latter be kept up unfailingly.

3. Now, just one more word to those who think it impossible to give up the accustomed mucus food (meat, bread, etc.). To those "unfortunate ones," I give this advice: Chew each bite of your food thoroughly as recommended by the American, Fletcher—in one word, "Fletcherize." Not that the fruit eaters should overlook this, but certainly the poison-laden "mucus-eaters" must do so, especially if they do not wish to sink into their graves all too soon.

The strong secretion of saliva in slow chewing decreases the formation of mucus and helps to prevent overeating. Of course, this group of individuals cannot expect to achieve in health and strength; retain youth and perseverance; physical and mental efficiency, as achieved by the faster and fruit eater! Once a person is healthy, in my sense of the word, through fasting and fruit diet (that is, free from mucus, slime, and germs) and continues on the fruit diet, they, of course, need not fast any longer; for only then will they find pleasure in eating that which they never dreamt of before. Only in this way will humans find the way to happiness, harmony, and the solution of all health problems. Only through following this diet can humans become want-free and get "nearest to divinity."

The Fundamental Cause of Growing Old and Ugly

THE MEANS FOUNDED IN NATURE FOR MAINTENANCE OF YOUTH AND BEAUTY

Following the previous general arguments to the effect that mucus is the main cause of disease and aging, there is only left to show in particular and on the various organs, in how far the mucus of culture food acts "beauty hindering" in the construction of the human body and produces symptoms of ugliness and age.

If, according to paradisiac primary laws, the lungs and skin would be given nothing but pure air and sun-electricity, and the stomach and bowels nothing but sun-food, (i.e., fruits), which are being digested almost without rest, secreting only mucusless, pasteless, and germless cellulose, there seems to be no reason why the tube system of the human body should become defective, weaken, age, and finally break down entirely. Instead of the living energy cells of the fruit, one eats "killed food," which biologically is meant for beasts of prey, i.e., food chemically changed by air-oxidation (decay), dead-boiled, and robbed of its energy. Mucus accumulates especially in the heating channel (stomach and bowels) of the tube machine, and slowly clogs up the channel and filters (glands). The sum total of this defilement causes chronic defects, makes one grow old, and is the main factor in the nature of all disease. Growing old, therefore, is actually a latent

27

disease, that is, a slow but constantly increasing disturbance in the operation of the motor of life.

The chemistry of victuals gives the most reliable proof that deformity and decomposition have their source mainly in the lack of minerals in boiled culture food.

If human ugliness as such, lost beauty, and symptoms of growing old can be made accountable for by wrong nourishment, then the theory of beauty and rejuvenation leads to a dietetic cure and a respective improvement of nourishment. But inasmuch as beauty, especially human beauty, cannot be absolutely defined, because everybody has a different taste, I can limit myself only to the main standards of aesthetic demands.

The white corpse-color of the light and sunless humans of culture cannot be considered beautiful, since it emanates mainly from the white corpse-color of the dead-boiled, wrong food. What wonderful color a person can get, who feeds on "bleeding" grapes, cherries, and oranges, and who systematically takes air baths and sunbaths, cannot be imagined by the modern artists of "pleinair-painting." Mucus, and at the same time lack of mineral matter, means as much as lack of color. Just compare the food tables of Dr. Konig and you will find that the mucusless food, the fruits and starchless, green-leaf vegetables, occupy the first place as regards their contents of necessary mineral matter, especially lime. The size of a person, i.e., the circumference of the skeleton, depends for instance mainly on the amount of lime contained in the food. The Japanese want to increase the size of their race by meat, thereby going from bad to worse. All the pining away of size, deformities of the bones, and faulty vision and decay of the teeth is due to lack of lime. Through the boiling of milk and vegetables in modern cooking, the lime content is being eliminated. The enormous poorness in minerals of cultured food, especially of the meat as compared with fruit, is responsible for the coming of a toothless human race, as predicted even by physicians, and which is not merely a phantom of imagination. And instead of by fruit, these stuffs are being substituted by an organic preparation. The human organism does not assimilate one single atom of mineral substance which has not transmigrated into a plant of fruit, i.e., which has not become organic. The most modern disfigurement, the obesity, has clouded up our aesthetic feeling in this regard so much that we even do not know any longer the limit of the normal. I personally do not even consider the physical culturist "man or woman of muscles of classic type" beautiful and as a standard for the ideal type of Germanic and Aryan races. Weight, shape, and especially circumference of body are too great. Every accumulation of fat is pathologic and in this measure unaesthetic. No animal living in freedom is upholstered with fat like our modern "weight lifters and strong men." The reason is simply too much food and too much fluid; relaxation and clogging of the entire system of vessels are the natural consequences. Grape sugar of the fruits and their nutritive salts are the right sources for a firm muscle-substance, by which a body disfattened and dismucused by fasting can be quickly rebuilt.

The stoutness of face and body are dangerously on the increase; it is ugly and certainly pathologic. It is a curious fact that in our supposedly enlightened age this accumulation of fat is considered not only beautiful, but even a sign of overabundant health, while the daily experience teaches that the slim, permanently youthful type possesses in every respect a greater force of resistance and generally reaches greater longevity.

I should like to be shown just one person of 90 or 100 years with such obesity, which today is pronounced as beautiful and healthy, and with which it is believed to fatten away tuberculosis. If fat people do not die in their best years through palpitation of the heart, apoplexy, or dropsy, they succumb to a slow emaciating and the desire for food decreases in spite of all artificial stimulations of the appetite. The skin, especially of the face, having been subjected to extreme tension, becomes foldy and wrinkly. It has lost its youthful elasticity on account of insufficient and unhealthy blood circulation, as well as lack of light and sun. And now this relaxation of the skin is being tried to be prevented by salves and powders applied externally! The distinction and beauty of the features: the pureness and healthy color of the complexion, the clearness and natural size of the eyes, the charm of the expression and the color of the lips, age and become ugly to the extent of the expression and color of the mucus in the bowels, which we have recognized above as the central depot from which all the symptoms of diseases, and therefore those of age, are being fed. The "beautiful roundness of cheeks," which at the same time increases the size of the nose, is nothing but a clogging up by mucus, which, as is well known, breaks out in case of a cold in the nose.

The Preservation of the Hair

REASONS FOR BECOMING BALD AND GRAY

I come now to the most important and most striking symptom of the growing-old: the falling out and getting gray of the hair, to which I must devote an entire section, because its appearance generally causes the first and greatest worry and pain over the coming of age, and because hitherto science has stood baffled in the face of this problem.

The modern cutting short of the feminine as well as the masculine hair on the head, and the alarming expansion and earliness of baldness have accustomed even an artistic eye so much to this appearance that we no longer become conscious of the fact of how seriously the aesthetic and harmonic figure of humans are disturbed by the voluntary and involuntary "hair decapitation." Humans who are not only intellectual, but also are an aesthetic product of nature, "the crown of creation," are being robbed of the splendid crown of their heads—the hair. They could be called "living skulls," these beardless, colorless, and expressionless heads of today! Just imagine the most beautiful woman with a pate! Where is the man or woman that would not turn away with horror? Or a fashion sport of today hewn in marble! In addition to that, the mustache, shaped geometrically and angular or trimmed off entirely; then the modern clothing which distinguishes itself from that of all the centuries by the greatest insipidity—and this we find beautiful; reasons for which the present-day man gets his beard removed and his hair cut down to a minimum length. The lack of beauty and therewith the unaesthetic appearance of hair and beard has become so general that in course of time the need of shaving and use of the clipper have come as a matter of course. In our time of equalization and all-leveling it is preferred, and rightfully so, to cut off these odor-, and so to speak, revelation-organs of inner humans instead of furnishing by ugly, disheveled, uneven, and hereditary morbid hair, a living proof for the descendants theory. Therewith, we can understand the maltreatment of the hair. The thought has practically given rise that the getting ugly of one organ or of the entire organism means its inner morbidness, i.e., nature reveals internal physiological disturbances of an organism through disharmony of shape and color. The seriously ill and dead organisms are its extremes. Doubters of my point of view and bad nature observers may here be reminded of the law of exception from the rule; and as regards humans, of the fact that neither hygienically nor aesthetically have we any imagination left of the ideal beauty and health of humans living under perfectly natural conditions. If the pleasure in the beautiful is a sentence in the favorable sense, then the displeasure felt by an aesthetic eye in looking upon the disharmony of shape and color must include to a certain degree the recognition of the pathologic.

Let us return to our subject. We know that medical science is powerless as regards baldness, and that cosmetics and chemistry of tonics have failed to produce even a single new hair.

I have already called the hair, especially of the human head, the odor-organs of the body, which are to conduct away the exhalations of the human body. Everybody knows that sweat is produced first of all on the head and in the armpits, and that with this sweat, especially on sick people, is connected a disagreeable odor. Dr. Jaeger calls disease somewhere "stench." This, with exceptions of course, seems to me correct insofar as I am able to pronounce, on the basis of many years' observation and experiments, the following fundamental uniform conception of disease:

> Disease is a fermentation and decay process of body substance or of surplus and unnatural food material, which in course of time has accumulated, especially in

32

the digestive organs, and which makes its appearance in the shape of mucus excretion.

That is, it means in the last instance nothing but the chemical decomposition, the decay, of cellular albumen. As is well known, this process is accompanied by stench, while nature combines the originating of new life with fragrance (the building of plants). Properly, humans in perfect health should exhale fragrance, particularly so with their hair. Poets are rightfully comparing humans with a flower and speak of the hair fragrance of woman. I, THEREFORE, RECOGNIZE IN THE HAIR OF THE HUMAN A VERY IMPORTANT ORGAN, WHICH ASIDE FROM PROTECTIVE AND WARMTH-REGULATING PURPOSES, HAS A HIGHLY INTERESTING AND USEFUL DESTINATION: to conduct away the exhalations, the odor of healthy and sick people, which reveal to experts and acute noses not only individual qualities but even certain disclosures as regards the inner state of health or sickness of a human. If the doctors have not by far recognized digestive disturbances with the microscopes and test glasses, there have yet been certain quacks who have been able to state by simple hair diagnosis the stench-producing inner process of decay—the disease. Why, there are numberless people today, still youthful and radiating health, with a breath like that of a sewer and who are wondering why their hair is falling out.

I have now arrived at the vital spot of my researches and observations.

First, one more word about the getting gray of the hair. It has been found that in hair that has become gray, the contents of air is increasing; and I am also of the opinion that this "air" consists probably of stinking gases, or at least is mixed with such. I recommend to a chemist with a "strong scent" to discover here the sulfurous acid, then the disappearance of the color of the hair will also have been explained, as it is a well-known fact that sulfur dioxide bleaches organic substances.

It now seems to me certain, not only theoretically, but also on the basis of my interesting experiments on my own body, that the principal cause of baldness can only be an internal one. If through these odor tubes or, so to speak, "gas chimneys of the head," there must be constantly discharged stinking, corroding gases, very probably impregnated with sulfur dioxide, instead of natural, fragrant odors, we must not be surprised if the hair together with its roots becomes deathly pale, dies off, and falls out. Herewith, I claim to have recognized the reason for baldness and to have shown the true way for its cure. I add that about 10 years ago, when I was afflicted with chronic inflammation of the kidneys combined with a high degree of nervousness, my hair had become very gray and fell out. After having been cured from this serious disease by a dietetic treatment, I saw that at the same time the gray hairs disappeared and that my hair grew into perfect profusion.

If, therefore, the main cause of baldness lies in the disturbance of digestion and interchange of matter, it can certainly be cured by regulation of these functions. It can be said that even the absolutely bald heads may again take hope on the basis of my discovery—after all the tonics have failed, and must fail. The reason is that the cause is not external and therefore cannot be got at externally. Whoever sees their hair falling out, or whoever is already bald and wishes to regenerate in this direction, may apply to me for advice. There is no general internal remedy, and whoever has understood me will appreciate that individualization is necessary in every case. On the basis of the influence of my doctrine of diet on digestion, and creation of clean, pure blood supplying the correct nourishment of the hair bed, I can at least guarantee a standstill of the falling out of hair, if my advice is followed correctly.

Thus, all symptoms of aging are latent disease, accumulation of mucus, and clogging-up by mucus. Everybody subjecting himself to a thorough restoring cure in case of any disease, by parting with the dead cells through mucusless diet and eventually fasting, rejuvenates himself simultaneously; and whoever submits to a rejuvenating cure deprives each and every disease of its foundation. Nobody wants to believe in this possibility. Yet, in each scientific dictionary you will find the theory that at the worst, one should die only of disturbance in the exchange of matter, i.e., constipation by mucus, so that life ought to end without any disease whatever. This would be the normal; but, alas, the exception—the disease has become the rule today.

IF ANYBODY WOULD LIVE FROM CHILDHOOD ON ABSOLUTELY MUCUSLESS FOOD AND FEED ON NOTHING BUT FRUIT, IT WOULD BE JUST AS CERTAIN THAT HE OR SHE COULD GROW NEITHER OLD NOR SICK. I have seen persons who through a mucusless cure have rejuvenated and become beautiful to such an extent that they could not be recognized. Since thousands of years, humanity dreams, imagines, and paints the fountain of youth and looks for it sentimentally to the stars in the suggestion.

Think of the amounts being expended for remedies for masculine weakness and impotence, for sterility—of course all in vain! And how easy it would be to help some people, especially through correct and nourishing food from the sun kitchen.

We cannot imagine with what beauty and faculties the paradisiacal "godlike" man and woman were gifted, what wonderful strong, clear voices they had! The beautification and strengthening of the voice; yes, the winning back of the lost voice is an amazing symptom in my cure and especially eloquent proof for the really grandiose effect of my system for the entire organism of the patient. I wish to refer here especially to the wonderful success of the cure submitted to by the Royal Bavarian Chamber Singer Heinrich Knote, Munich, under my directions, whose voice had improved to the amazement of the entire musical world.

Increasing Longevity

In the previous chapters, I have quoted the clogging-up by mucus as being the reason for disease and aging. I have also proved the possibility of resubstitution of dead cells. In view of the latter fact, it cannot be denied that the entire standstill of the human motor can be delayed for a long, long time if the body is being built up and maintained by living sun food from childhood on. At any rate, the body thus nourished is far ahead of that of the wrong food and "all-eater," in that its building material is much more durable. In the right way of living, the exchange of matter takes place to a much lesser degree; likewise the stress on the inner organs, especially the heart and the stomach. In the performance of greatest efforts, the mucusless organism has not nearly the pulse frequency of a "much-eater." Merely through this saving of energy, it is possible to mathematically figure out and prove an advantage as regards longevity. But can we perhaps even solve by this all-explaining mucus constipation the last of all mysteries—death?

In life-endangering injuries and afflictions, the brain and the heart are the organs whose disturbance of function finally ends with death. We can say that in most diseases death takes place through additional development of heart illness. As regards this, science has not by far spoken its last word, but we can say that the clogging-up of the blood vessels of the heart and the destruction of the tender heart nerves through permanent re-poisoning of the blood is the final cause of death in all chronic diseases. Likewise, the clogging up of the tender blood vessels in the brain and an eventual bursting of same (apoplexy), as well as any other entire clogging-up of vessels to a standstill of all functions of life, produce death. Of course, other circumstances also play a part in it, for instance, insufficient supply of air in case of disease of the lungs. Science also mentions the excessive appearance of the white blood corpuscles as the reason for death. This process of disease is regarded as a disease in itself, and called "Leukemia"—white bloodedness; but more proper in my opinion: more mucus than blood. Many other reasons are given for the cause of death.

If, perchance, a disease cannot be put into any of the better-defined registers, it is given the name of "cachexy," which sounds very wise but means bad conditions of nourishment, decay. I now ask, what is really the killing poison? Modern medical science gives the bacilli as the cause for most of the diseases, thus showing that it also has the idea of a common fundamental factor for all diseases, the aging, and death, and undoubtedly a large part of all diseases and their consequences (death) are due to the bacilli. My experimental proof that mucus is the fundamental and main factor differs from the bacillus theory only in that just this mucus is the bed, the pre-condition, the primary.

The excessive appearance of the white blood corpuscles, i.e., of the white dead mucus, as compared with the red sugar and iron substances, is becoming dangerous to life. Red colored and sweet is the visible token of life and love; white, pale, colorless, bitter the token of disease and overwhelming by mucus, the slow dying-away of the individual.

The death struggle or agony can only be regarded as a last crisis, a last effort of the organism to excrete mucus, a last fight of the still-living cells against the dead ones and their death poisons. If the white, dead cells—the mucus in the blood—gain the upper hand, there takes place not only a mechanical clogging-up in the heart, but also a chemical reformation, a decline, a total poisoning, a sudden decay of the entire blood supply—and the machine stops short. "It has pleased God Almighty"; "we bend our knees before the mysterious power of death"—thus we speak with resignation.

PART II

Complete Instructions for Fasting

Most diseases are due to wrong eating habits, incorrect food combinations, acidulous foods, and the commercial foods of present-day civilization. How to overcome the results of these errors that the majority of us ignorantly inflict upon ourselves will be taught in the following pages.

For thousands of years, fasting has been recognized as Nature's supreme curative measure. But the art of when, why, and how to fast has been lost by those living in present-day civilization with a very few exceptions. The body must have good, nourishing food—is the battle cry of today. But just what is good, nourishing food?

The unfortunate sufferers go the rounds of the various schools of therapeutics, some of them deliberate fakirs—others unknowingly ignorant, but in the majority of cases groping darkly and in vain for the truth. And the unfortunate part of it all is that they die before they learn the truth. Religious evangelists and divine healers have the advantage of giving Nature a chance—prescription "specialists," scientific surgery—serum injectors and vaccine inoculators are the real offenders of an outraged nature. And so it resolves itself into a case of "blind leading the blind." How simple it is to receive instructions from Nature. Watch the animals heal themselves in time

39

of illness—without the use of so-called scientific medicine. This, then, is the supreme secret of Mother Nature's self-healing.

In these chapters, we intend showing why it is necessary to use cooked foods as well as natural foods to properly balance your diet. We will also explain the causes of fermentation and gas-producing foods.

Rational Fasting for Physical, Mental, and Spiritual Rejuvenation

It is significant for our time of degeneration that fasting, by which I mean living without solid and liquid food, is still a problem as a leading factor for the average human, as well as for the orthodox medical doctor. Even naturopathy required a few decades in its development to take up Nature's only, universal and omnipotent "remedy" of healing. It is further significant that fasting is still considered as a "special" kind of cure, and due to some truly "marvelous" results here and there, it has quite recently become a worldwide fad. Some expert Nature-cure advocators plan out general "prescriptions" of fasting and how to break a fast, regardless of your condition or the cause from which you are a sufferer.

On the other hand, fasting is so feared and misrepresented that the average person actually considers you a fool if you miss a few meals when sick, thinking you will starve to death, when in reality you are being cured. They fail to understand the difference between fasting and starvation. The medical doctor in general endorses and, in fact, teaches such foolish beliefs regarding Nature's only foundational law of all healing and "curing."

Whatever has been designed and formulated to eliminate the disease matters and designated as "natural treatments" without having at least some restriction or change in diet, or fasting, is a fundamental disregard of the truth concerning the cause of disease.

Have you ever thought what the lack of appetite means when sick? And that animals have no doctors, and no drug stores, and no sanitariums, and no machinery to heal them? Nature demonstrates and teaches by that example that there is only one disease and that one is caused through eating—and, therefore, every disease, whatsoever it may be named by humans, is and can be healed by one "remedy" only—by doing the direct opposite of the cause—by the compensation of the wrong—i.e., reducing the quantity of food, or fasting. The reason so many, and especially long-fasting, cures have failed and continue to fail is due to the ignorance which still exists, regarding what is going on in the body during a fast—an ignorance still existing even in the minds of naturopaths and fasting experts up to the present date.

I dare say there may not be another person in history who has studied, investigated, tested, and experimented on fasting as much as I did. There is no other expert at present, as far as I know, who conducted so many fasting cures on the most severe cases, as I did. I opened the first special sanitarium in the world for fasting, combined with the mucusless diet, and fasting is an essential part of my *Mucusless Diet Healing System*. I have likewise made four public scientific tests of fastings of 21, 24, 32, and 49 days, respectively, as a scientific demonstration. The latter test is the **world's record of a fast conducted under a strict scientific supervision of government officials.**

You may therefore believe me when I teach something new and instructive about what actually happens in the body during a fast. You have learned that the body must be first considered as a machine, a mechanism made of rubber-like material that has been overexpanded during its entire life through overeating. Therefore, the functioning of the organism is continually obstructed by an unnatural overpressure of the blood and on the tissues. As soon as you stop eating, this overpressure is rapidly relieved, the avenues of the circulation contract, the blood becomes more concentrated, and the superfluous water is eliminated. This goes on for the first few days and you may even feel fine; but then the obstructions of the circulation become greater because the diameter of the avenues become smaller, and the blood must circulate through many parts of the body, especially in the tissues at and around the symptom, against sticky mucus, pressed out and dissolved from the inside walls. In other words, the bloodstream must overcome, dissolve, and carry with itself mucus and poisons for elimination through the kidneys.

When you fast, you eliminate first and at once the primary obstructions of wrong and too much eating. This results in your feeling relatively good or possibly even better than when eating; but as previously explained, you bring new, secondary obstructions from your own waste in the circulation and you feel miserable. You and everyone else blame the lack of food. The next day you can notice with certainty mucus in the urine, and when the quantity of waste taken in the circulation is eliminated, you will undoubtedly feel fine, even stronger than ever before. So it is a well-known fact that a faster can feel better and is actually stronger on the twentieth day than on the fifth or sixth day—certainly a tremendous proof that vitality does not depend primarily on food, but rather from an unobstructed circulation. (See Lesson 5 of my *Mucusless Diet Healing System.*) The smaller the amount of "O" (obstruction), the greater "P" (air pressure), and therefore "V" (vitality).

Through the above enlightening explanation, you see that fasting is first, a negative proposition to relieve the body from direct obstructions of solid, most unnatural foods; second, that it is a mechanical process of elimination by contracting tissues pressing out mucus, causing friction and obstruction in the circulation.

The following are examples of vitality from "P" Power, air-pressure alone:

One of my first fasters, a relatively healthy vegetarian, walked 45 miles in the mountains on his twenty-fourth fast day.

A friend, 15 years younger, and I walked 56 HOURS CONTINUALLY after a 10-day fast.

A German physician, a specialist in fasting cures, published a pamphlet entitled "Fasting, the Increase of Vitality." He learned the same fact that I did, but he does not know why and how, and vitality therefore remained mysterious for him.

If you drink only water during a fast, the human mechanism cleanses itself the same as though you would press out a dirty watery sponge; but the dirt in this instance is sticky mucus, and in many

43

cases pus and drugs, which must pass through the circulation until it is so thoroughly dissolved that it can pass through the fine structure of the "physiological sieve" called kidneys.

Building a Perfect Body through Fasting

As long as the waste is in the circulation, you feel miserable during a fast; as soon as it is through the kidneys, you feel fine. Two or three days later and the same process repeats itself. It must now be clear to you why conditions change so often during a fast; it must now be clear to you why it is possible for you to feel unusually better and stronger on the twentieth day than on the fifth, for instance.

But this entire cleansing work through continued contracting of the tissue (becoming lean) must be done by and with the original, old blood composition of the patient; and consequently, a long fast, especially a too-long fast, may become in fact a crime if the sick organism is too greatly clogged up by waste. Fasters who died from too long a fast did not die from lack of food, but actually suffocated in and with their own waste. I made this statement years ago. More clearly expressed: the immediate cause of death is not a poverty of blood in vital substances, but from too much obstruction. "O" (obstruction) becomes as great as or even greater than "P" (air pressure), and the body mechanism is at its "death point."

I GAVE ALL OF MY FASTERS LEMONADE WITH A TRACE OF HONEY OR BROWN SUGAR FOR LOOSENING AND THINNING THE MUCUS IN THE CIRCULATION. Lemon juice and fruit acids of all kinds neutralize the stickiness of mucus and pus (acid paste cannot be used).

If a patient has ever taken drugs over their entire life period,— which are stored up in the body like the waste from food—their condition might easily become serious or even dangerous when these poisons enter the circulation, when a person takes their first fast. Palpitation of the heart, headaches, nervousness may set in, and especially insomnia. I saw patients eliminate drugs they had taken as long as 40 years before. Symptoms such as described above are blamed on the fast by everybody and especially doctors.

How Long Should One Fast?

Nature answers this question in the animal kingdom with a certain cruelty—"fast until you are either healed or dead!" In my estimation, 50 to 60 percent of the so-called "healthy" men of today and 80 to 90 percent of the seriously chronic sick would die from their latent diseases through a long fast.

How long one should fast cannot be definitely stated at all, in advance, even in cases where the condition of the patient is known. When and how to break the fast is determined by noting carefully how conditions change during the fast—you now understand that the fast should be broken as soon as you notice that the obstructions are becoming too great in the circulation, and the blood needs new, vital substance to resist and neutralize the poisons.

Change your ideas regarding the claim, "the longer you fast the better the cure." You may now readily understand why. Humans are the sickest animals on earth. No other animal has violated the laws of eating as much as humans; no other animal eats as wrongly as them.

Here is the point where human intelligence can correctively assist in the self-healing process by the following adjustments that embrace the *Mucusless Diet Healing System*:

First—Prepare for an easier fast by a gradually changing diet toward a mucusless diet, and natural herbal laxatives and enemas.

Second—Change shorter fasts periodically with some eating days of cleansing "mucus-poor" and mucusless diet.

Third—Be particularly careful if the patient used much drugs, especially if a mercury or saltpeter, oxide of silver (taken for venereal diseases) have been used, in which case a long, slowly changing, preparative diet is advisable.[2]

An "expert's" suggestion to fast until the tongue is clean caused many troubles with "fanatical" fasters, and I personally know of one death. You may be surprised when I tell you that I had to cure patients from the ill effects of too long a fast. The reason will be clear later.

In spite of the above, every cure, and especially every cure of diet, should start with a 2- or 3-day fast. Every patient can do this without any harm, regardless of how seriously sick they may be. First a laxative and then an enema daily, makes it easier as well as harmless.

How to Break a Fast

I consider the knowledge of how to break a fast of the utmost importance.

The right food after a fast itself. At the same time, it depends entirely upon the condition of the patient and very much upon the length of the fast. You may learn from the results of the two extreme cases, both of which ended fatally—not from the fast, but from the first wrong meal—just why this knowledge is so important.

A one-sided meat eater suffering from diabetes broke his fast, which lasted about a week, by eating dates, and died from the effects. A person of over 60 years of age fasted 28 days (too long); his first meal of vegetarian foods consisting mainly of boiled potatoes. A necessary operation showed that the potatoes were kept in the contracted intestines by thick, sticky mucus so strong that a piece had to be cut off and the patient died shortly after the operation.

---

[2] Mercury is no longer used to treat venereal diseases, although mercury-based dental amalgam fillings continue to the present day in the midst of much controversy. If you had, or have, mercury fillings, you will want to be careful as you begin to use the *Mucusless Diet Healing System*. For support and guidance in safely confronting mercury-related issues using the mucusless diet, it is advisable to seek assistance from an expert *Mucusless Diet Healing System* practitioner. Also be sure to read the *Mucusless Diet Healing System*.

In the first case, the terrible poisons loosened in the stomach of this one-sided meat eater during his fast, when mixed with the concentrated fruit sugar of the dates, caused at once so great a fermentation with carbonic acid gases and other poisons that the patient could not stand the shock. The correct advice would be: First a laxative, such as a preparation consisting of harmless herbs; later raw and cooked starchless vegetables, a piece of rough bran bread toast. Sauerkraut is to be recommended in such cases. No fruits should be eaten for a long time after the fast has been broken. The patient should have been prepared for the fast by a longer transition diet.

In the second case, the patient fasted entirely too long for a person of his age without proper preparation.

Through these two very instructive examples you may see how individually different the advice must be, and how wrong it is to make up general suggestions concerning how to break a fast.

Important Rules for the Faster

TO BE CAREFULLY STUDIED AND MEMORIZED

What can be said in general, and what I teach is new and different from the average fasting experts, and is as follows:

1. The first meal and the menus for a few days after a fast must be of a laxative effect, and not of nourishing value as mostly all others think.

2. The sooner the first meal passes through the body the more efficiently it carries out the loosened mucus and poisons of the intestines and the stomach.

3. If no good stool is experienced after 2 or 3 hours—help with laxatives and enemas. Whenever I fasted, I always experienced a good bowel movement at least 1 hour after eating, and at once felt fine. After breaking a long fast I spent more time on the toilet than in bed the following night—and that was as it should be.

While sojourning in Italy many years ago, I drank about two quarts of fresh grape juice after a fast. At once, I experienced a watery diarrhea set in foaming mucus. Almost immediately after, I experienced a feeling of such unusual strength that I easily performed the knee-bending and arm-stretching exercise 326 times. This removal so thoroughly of obstructions, taking place after a fast of a few days, increased "P"—vitality at once! You will have to experience a similar sensation to believe me, and then you will agree with my formula, "Vitality equals Power minus Obstructions," and you will realize the absurdity of making up scientific nourishing menus for health and efficiency.

4. The longer the fast the more efficiently the bowels perform after it is over.

5. The best laxative foods after a fast are fresh sweet fruits; best of all are cherries and grapes, then a little soaked or stewed prunes. These fruits must not be used after a meat eater's first fast, but only for people who have lived for a certain time on mucusless or at least mucus-poor foods—the "transition diet."

6. In the average case, it is advisable to break the fast with raw and cooked starchless vegetables; stewed spinach has an especially good effect.

7. If the first meal does not cause any unpleasantness, you may eat as much as you can. Eating only a small quantity of food for the first 2 or 3 days without experiencing a bowel movement—owing to the small amount of food taken—(another wrong advice given by "experts")—is dangerous.

8. If you are in the proper condition so that you can start eating with fruits, and you have no bowel movement after about an hour, then eat more or eat a vegetable meal as suggested above, eat until you bring out the waste accumulated during the fast with your stool, after eating the first meal.

Rules during the Fast

1. Clean the lower intestines as well as you can with enemas, at least every other day.

2. Before starting a longer fast, take a laxative occasionally and by all means the day before you start the fast.

3. If possible, remain in the fresh air, day and night.

4. Take a walk, exercise, or some other physical work only when you feel strong enough to do it; if tired and weak, rest and sleep as much as you can.

5. On days when you feel weak, and you will experience such days when the waste is in the circulation, you will find that your sleep is restless and disturbed, and you may experience bad dreams. This is caused through the poisons passing through the brain. Doubt—loss of faith will arise in your mind; then take this lesson and read it over and over, as well as the other fasting chapters, and especially Lesson 5 of my *Mucusless Diet Healing System* book. Don't forget that you are, parenthetically speaking, lying on Nature's operating table; the most wonderful of all operations that could be performed; and without the use of a knife! If any extraordinary sensation occurs due to the drugs that are now in circulation, take an enema at once, lie down, and if necessary break the fast, but not with fruits.

6. Whenever you arise after lying down, do it slowly; otherwise you may become dizzy. The latter condition is not serious, but you had better avoid it in this manner. It caused me a considerable fear in the beginning, and I know a number of fasters and strict eaters who gave up when they experienced this sensation—lost their faith forever.

Fasting Drinks

The "fanatic" fasting enthusiast drinks only water. He or she thinks it best to avoid any trace of food whatever. I CONSIDER A LIGHT LEMONADE WITH A LITTLE HONEY OR BROWN SUGAR OR A LITTLE FRUIT JUICE THE BEST. Drink as often as you care to during the day, but in general, not more than two to three quarts a day. The less you drink the more aggressive the fast works.

As a change, vegetable juice made from cooked starchless vegetables is very good during a longer fast. Raw tomato juice, etc., is also good. But if fruit juice, for example, orange juice, is used during a longer fast, be extremely careful because the fruit juices may cause the poisons to become loosened too rapidly without causing a bowel movement. I know a number of such fruit and fruit-juice fasts which failed completely because all mucus and all poisons loosened too fast and too much at one time, disturbs all organs too greatly when in the circulation, and have to be eliminated only through the circulation without the aid of bowel movements.

Morning Fast or Non-Breakfast Plan

The worst of all eating habits nowadays is to stuff the stomach with food early in the morning. In European countries, excepting England, no one takes a regular meal for breakfast; it is generally a drink of some kind with bread only.

The only time that a human does not eat for 10 or 12 hours is while they are asleep during the night. As soon as his or her stomach is free from food, the body starts the eliminating process of a fast; therefore, encumbered people feel miserable and have a coated tongue upon awakening in the morning. They have no appetite at all, yet they crave food, eat it, and feel better—WHY?

Another Mystery Revealed

This is one of the greatest problems I solved, and is one that has puzzled all "experts" who believe it is the food itself. As soon as you refill the stomach with food, THE ELIMINATION IS STOPPED and you feel better! I must say that this secret which I discovered is undoubtedly the explanation of why eating became a habit and is no longer what nature intended it should be, i.e., a satisfaction, a compensation of nature's need of food.

This habit of eating, striking all civilized humankind and now physiologically explained, involves and proves the saying I coined long ago—"Life is a tragedy of nutrition." The more waste that humans accumulate, the more they must eat to stop the elimination. I had patients who had to eat several times during the night to be able to sleep again. In other words, they had to put food in the stomach to avoid the digestion of mucus and poisons, accumulated there.

Short Fasts and the Non-Breakfast Plan

During my experience with thousands of fasters, I had patients that had to eat several times during the night in order to sleep again. The reason is very apparent. Let me cite an example. Upon awakening, you perhaps feel fine—but instead of getting up, you remain in bed and fall asleep again—have a bad dream, and actually feel miserable upon awakening the second time. You can understand the exact reason for this.

As soon as you get up, walk around, or do something, the body is in an entirely different condition than during the sleep. The elimination is slowed down, the energy being used elsewhere.

If eating breakfast is eliminated from your daily menus, you will probably experience some harmless sensation such as headaches for the first 1 or 2 days; but after that, you will feel much better, work better, and enjoy your luncheon better than ever. Hundreds of severe cases have been cured by the "non-breakfast fast" alone, without important changes in diet, proving that the habit of a full breakfast meal is the worst of all and most injurious.

It is advisable and really of great advantage to allow the patient to have the same drink for breakfast that he or she is accustomed to; if he or she craves coffee, let them continue their drink of coffee, but absolutely no SOLID food! Later on, replace the coffee with a warm vegetable juice, and still later change to lemonade. This change should be made gradually for the average mixed eater.

The 24-Hour Fast or One-Meal-a-Day Plan

As with the breakfast fast, you can heal more severe cases with the 24-hour fast, for in cases of deep, chronic encumbrance and drugs, it is a careful, preliminary step to the necessary longer fasts. The best time to eat is in the afternoon, say, 3:00 or 4:00 p.m.

If the patient is on the mucusless or transition diet, let him eat the fruits first—(fruits should always be eaten first)—and after an elapse of 15 or 20 minutes eat the vegetables; but all should be eaten within an hour so that it is to say, one meal.

Fasting When Used in Connection with the *Mucusless Diet Healing System*

As I have stated before, I am no longer in favor of long fasts. In fact, it may become criminal to let a patient fast for 30 or 40 days on water—contracting the avenues of circulation—which are continually filling up more and more with mucus and by dangerous old drugs and poisons, and at the same time rotten blood from his or her old "stock"—in fact, actually starving from necessary vital food elements. No one can stand a fast of that kind without disadvantage or without harming vitality.

If fasting is to be used at all, then start at first with the non-breakfast plan; then follow with the 24-hour fast for a while; then gradually increase up to 3-, 4-, or 5-day fasts, eating between fasts for 1, 2, 3, or 4 days a mucusless diet, combined individually as an elimination adjustment, and at the same time supplying and rebuilding the body continually with and by the best elements contained in and found only in mucusless foods.

Through such intermittent fasts the blood is gradually improved, regenerated, can more easily tolerate the poisons and waste, and the patient is able at the same time to dissolve and eliminate "disease deposits" from the deepest tissues of the body; deposits that no doctor ever dreamed existed, and that no other method of healing has ever discovered or can remove.

This, then, is the *Mucusless Diet Healing System*, with fasting an essential part of it.

Fasting in Cases of Acute Disease

"Hunger Cures—Wonder Cures" was the title of the first fasting book I ever read. It gave the experiences of a country doctor, in which he said, "No feverish, acute disease must nor can end with death if nature's instinctive command to stop eating through lack of appetite is followed."

It is insanity to give food to a pneumonia patient with a high fever, for instance. Having had an unusual contraction of the lung tissues by a "cold," the pressed-out mucus goes into the circulation and produces an unusual heat-fever. The human engine, already through heat at the bursting point, becomes more heated through partaking of solid food, meat broth, etc. (good nourishing foods).

Air baths taken in the room, enemas, laxatives, and cool lemonade would save the lives of thousands of young men who are now daily permitted to die, the innocent victims of pneumonia, or other acute diseases—due to the stubborn ignorance of doctors and so-called highly civilized people.

Fasting for Spiritual Rebirth through
the Superior Fast

All experts except myself believe that you live from your own flesh during a fast. You know now that what they call metabolism—"metabolize your own flesh when you fast"—is simply the elimination of waste.

The Indian "fakir," the greatest fakir in the world today, is nothing but skin and bones. I learned that the cleaner you are, the easier it is to fast and the longer you can stand it. In other words, in a body free from all waste and poisons and when no solid foods are taken, the human body functions for the first time in its life without obstructions. The elasticity of the entire tissue system, and of the internal organs, especially of the spongy lungs, work with an entirely different vibration and efficiency than ever before, by air alone, and without the slightest obstructions. Stated differently: "V" equals "P," and if you simply supply the "engine" with the necessary water that is used up, you ascend into a higher state of physical, mental, and spiritual condition. I call that the "superior fast."

If your blood "stock" is formed from eating the foods I teach, your brain will function in a manner that will surprise you. Your former life will take on the appearance of a dream, and for the first time in your existence, your conscience awakens to a real self-consciousness.

Your mind, your thinking, your ideals, your aspirations, and your philosophy change fundamentally in such a way as to beggar description.

Your soul will shout for joy and triumph over all misery of life leaving it all behind you. For the first time, you will feel a vibration of vitality through your body—like a slight electric current—that shakes you delightfully.

You will learn and realize that fasting and superior fasting (and not volumes of psychology and philosophy) is the real and only key to a superior life, to the revelation of a superior world, and to the spiritual world.

All of my "experiments" were made on my own person before being used on patients. My health experiments began while still holding a professorship in Baden-Baden, Germany, where I had become "incurably ill." My complete restoration to health—to what was probably the most perfect state of health of anyone living in our Western civilization today, was an interesting adventure of finding the fundamental laws of nature during my pursuit of health. I found that the body normalizes itself if properly cleansed of toxic wastes and supplied with proper nutrition. "MUCUS" is the keynote of the misunderstanding. I have consistently and definitely proven that a mucusless diet, coupled with the wise use of fasting and observing the basic laws of physiology, is the "magic wand" by which our present-day civilization will be afforded a new lease on life. I contend that all disease, regardless of its "scientific" name, or the symptoms accompanying it consists of constitutional encumbrance of waste material known as "foreign matter." Nature continually attempts to eliminate this disease-producing waste encumbrance and to stop the source of it. My method of restoration performs exactly the same in the human body as instinctive self-healing does in the animal kingdom. The disease producing material is partially digested, decaying, semi-liquid generally known as "mucus." Everyone living on today's accepted mixed diet consisting of starchy vegetables, grains, and meat is more or less clogged up with "mucus,"—whether sick or not!

Conclusion

While I have conducted thousands of fasting cures, any number of people has been helped by simply changing their present dietary habits. The sudden change of diet causes disturbances even in an entirely healthy person. For this reason, a change made too rapidly may become dangerous, and a complete knowledge is therefore essential.

To relieve and avoid any disturbance of health and at the same time to replace the old "tidbit" enjoyments by new and better ones can be accomplished if one follows my transition diet. Changing from meat eating to a strictly vegetarian or fruitarian diet always results in a more vigorous feeling for the first few days; then weakness, great fatigue, possibly headaches, and palpitation of the heart set in.

Fruit, being the only natural food, loosens and dissolves the mucus, poisons, and toxemias, and the penned up filth and morass of overfeeding is passed out through the circulating blood. The dead, decayed tissues are pushed aside to make room for the new, living food substances, and for the time being the patient loses the change-of-matter balance. The elimination of poison through the circulating blood causes more or less disturbance of health. And unless you are thoroughly convinced of the efficacy of the natural diet, your friends will dissuade you from further attempts to cleanse the body and will urge an interruption of internal purification in order to save you from what they believe will result seriously; and you will soon become lean, the face will appear haggard and drawn, and a general depression of feeling may overtake you. This, then, is the healing crisis and if understandingly carried on will result in hoped-for good health. I divide all foods into two kinds.

1. Mucus-forming foods.

2. Non-mucus-forming foods.

Under the first heading, we find meat, eggs, fats, milk and all by-products made therefrom, dried beans, dried peas, lentils, and ALL STARCHY FOODS.

The second classification embraces: all non-starchy green vegetables and all kinds of fruits. There are certain vegetables and fruits that contain more or less starch, and should be given the place of secondary importance in the dietary.

Begin the transition with as much mucusless foods as possible and as little mucus-forming foods as possible. I call, this a mucus-lean diet. The next step towards health is the MUCUSLESS DIET, which means a combination of starchless vegetables and fruits. With the help of this transition diet and some knowledge by the individual to choose and combine rightly, the greatest and most important truth of life is revealed to him. The miscalled strength that we experience after meat eating is nothing but stimulation, for there is no nourishment for humans in meat: hardening of the arteries, in which fatty, plaque-shaped particles are deposited on the blood vessel walls. They build up a choking lining; in time, they may calcify and harden; high blood pressure often results. This kind of hardening of the arteries is the chief villain in death and disability. Heart attacks, arthritis, and diseases of senility stem from this same cause. The meat-eating animals will die on cooked meats without blood and bones! And rats soon die on an exclusive diet of white flour.

My mucus theory—now a proven fact—has been more and more recognized. It has withstood the test with enormous success and today has a platform that NATURAL TREATMENT AND DIET IS THE MOST PERFECT AND SUCCESSFUL SYSTEM OF HEALING KNOWN.

Nothing is easier than making promises merely by saying words—and nothing is more difficult than actually living up to these easily made promises day after day! What you promise today must be renewed and redecided tomorrow. For you, and no one else but you, must decide the "want to live." Ehret's health teachings, based on a natural diet over the years that lie ahead, must be followed. You will soon find life more desirable and you will enter with joyous gusto into things you formerly feared! A whole new vista will be opened to you!

Suffering humanity may now have the means of not only relieving but also PREVENTING disease, through *Rational Fasting* and the *Mucusless Diet* and developing an improved race of people that need never know what diseased conditions are. And my most fervent hope is that it will bring about a better-civilized humanity.

May this book serve all readers seeking after truth, regardless of its source; may it especially serve the sick, and encourage those worrying about the loss of their youth and the first sign of old age. And may this book find an increasingly larger audience who will accept and follow the truths it teaches—for fasting is not a fad but a definite cure, which must eventually establish itself in a permanent first place to the benefit of all humankind.

SECTION II

HEALTH AND HAPPINESS THROUGH FASTING:
When, Why, Where, and How to Fast

By Fred S. Hirsch

FASTING requires much more knowledge than the average health-seeker considers necessary. Hopefully, this article will help convince you that through fasting lies the road to health and happiness. Few individuals pay much attention to the underlying causes of human illness or the vital problems of what food is best for human consumption; and as a result, we innocently contribute to our own miseries and ailments through over-indulgence in eating incompatible food combinations; i.e., meat, alcoholic stimulants, dairy products, and starchy foods, excessive worry, tension, and overwork are all contributing factors.

FASTING must first be recognized as Nature's way of healing all ills, and while not a "cure-all" for every known ailment, total fasting makes it possible for Nature in her desperate and continuous effort to remove and expel the foreign matter and disease-producing toxemic wastes from the body, thereby correcting the faults of wrong living and improper diet.

FASTING may not be adapted to everyone, under every condition, but fortunately, fasting can prove acceptable to the great majority. Nature alone possesses the true healing power and our body

65

can therefore be designated a "self-curative" organism. For centuries past, we have been taught to look upon illness, "disease," as some deliberate affliction visited upon us—whether deserved or not—whereas in truth it is actually Nature's "housecleaning" effort! When this truism finally becomes recognized, and Nature, the great healer, is permitted to carry on, you will note a vast improvement in your health. Suppressing ailments and symptoms of pain through use of sedative and pain-relieving drugs must eventually result in the illness becoming chronic. During the course of a lifetime, toxemic wastes are continually being discharged, and it is claimed that the body and all vital organs have been renewed many times. Correcting wrong dietetic habits will permit the body to take advantage of this natural phenomenon and build clean healthy tissue! Only through a total fast can this be satisfactorily brought about. Voluntary abstinence from food for restoring normal bodily vigor was instinctive with primitive humans. Start fasting 1 or 2 days, drinking water only, to which a few drops of lemon or lime juice has been added, especially if distilled water is used. At about 4:00 or 5:00 in the afternoon, break the fast with a light laxative or enema. You will be shocked at the amount of waste that is now being thrown off almost immediately. This mass of previously uneliminated waste was poisoning your bloodstream circulation continuously. This should help convince you that here is the way—and the only way—to health!

It is the height of folly to expect modern "miracle drugs" to do more than to temporarily suppress the aches and pains of "disease." Because of the sedative ability of the narcotic drug to deaden the inflamed nerves and tissues for a few hours at most, Nature's "warning signals" are thereby ruthlessly disregarded! Arnold Ehret truthfully claims that "the basic cause of all latent disease of humans, whatever its official name may be, is a clogged-up tissue system of uneliminated, unused, and undigested food substances. Disease is still a mystery to every doctor who fails or deliberately refuses to understand and recognize these simple facts!" Disease consists of a "foreign matter" that has weight and that must be eliminated from the body before the patient can hope to get well. Every sick person must, therefore, go through the healing process of a "cleansing" so that the body may have the opportunity of eliminating the sticky "mucus," which has been stored in the tissues or held in the pockets

66

of the intestines for years and which interferes with the proper digestive and blood-building functions. Unfortunately, fasting is so feared by the average individual that they actually believe starvation will result through missing a few meals—when in reality they are being helped; and many practitioners fail to grasp, or fully understand, that there is a vast difference existing between fasting and starvation. A sure proof of the efficacy of fasting is to discontinue all food intake, with the exception of water, for a day or two. Note how the tongue (being an organ of elimination) becomes thickly coated with mucus. The odor of decaying foods is on your breath and the bowel eliminations become offensive. Probably for the first time, the body has now been given an opportunity of eliminating the overabundance of stored up wastes and encumbrances clogging up the tissues! Having assured yourself of the desirability of ridding your body of unwanted waste and encumbrances, the remedy consists of a series of short fasts—each fast to be followed by a "cleansing diet" of fruits and green-leaf vegetables, eaten either in their natural or cooked state. This "cleansing program" must be continued just so long as complete recovery to normal health is absent.

How Long Should One Fast

Every person has an individual problem—age of patient, nature of the illness, amount and type of drugs previously used. In fact, so many considerations need be given full recognition of this subject that the list would be endless. Fasting is Nature's oldest, yet least expensive and in our opinion best, method of treating disease. In fact, fasting can be considered the cornerstone of natural healing, and its value without equal. How long one should fast becomes important since long fasts of 30 to 50 days could become dangerous unless properly conducted and supervised by a knowledgeable authority. It is therefore wisest for the faster to adopt a series of short fasts, i.e., 2 or 3 days of each week, gradually increasing the length of each succeeding fast a day or more if necessary, but not to exceed more than a week of total fast at one time. This will enable the chronically ill body to gradually and slowly eliminate these toxic-waste materials responsible for their illness without seriously affecting normal body functioning; after which, a corrected mode of living will restore the individual to a virile, vigorous state of health. Fasting for overcoming both acute and chronic ailments is centuries old—dating back to the beginning of life itself. No claim is made that fasting is necessarily a pleasant experience, yet the faster often receives blessed relief from physical pain, plus self-satisfaction, in the knowledge that the fast might eventually result in complete cessation of all pain and, hopefully, a return to normalcy! Primarily, a fast is undertaken for a good reason—the individual is desirous of correcting and overcoming illness, or a depleted loss of vital power that has already manifested itself threatens to become chronic—so the answer to "how long should one fast" becomes clear—i.e., continue the short fasts until the illness has been overcome and disease no longer exists! This suggestion, of course, refers directly to the length of time that the series of "shorter fasts," as previously outlined, are to be continued.

Why to Fast

The search for health goes on unceasingly, and while fasting has helped untold thousands of sufferers to regain normal health, it is essential that we must know when, how, and why to fast in order that we might receive the greater amount of physical and mental benefit.

Arnold Ehret in his *Mucusless Diet Healing System* tells us, "Every disease, no matter what name it may be known by in medical science, is CONSTIPATION, i.e., a clogging-up of the entire pipe system of the human body." Please note that Ehret uses the word "constipation" to apply to "a clogging-up (a constipation) of the entire human pipe system" and not merely a "bowel evacuation," the ordinarily accepted usage of the word. They refer specifically to the accumulation of waste toxic matters in the tissues and in the bloodstream, the lungs, kidneys, bladder, stomach, intestinal tract—in fact, every organ of the entire body. And since in Ehret's opinion, 99.9 percent of all ailments directly result from the same causes, he aptly refers to all common ailments as "the one-ness of disease." Hence, the method of correction of the common cold, bronchitis, asthma, sinusitis, or tuberculosis, can best be accomplished through fasting, since in his opinion all ailments are the direct result of a "clogged up," overloaded mucus condition brought about through wrong dietetic habits—i.e., the overeating of "mucus-forming" types of food. The simple remedial expedient is to discontinue doing that which was the original cause of the condition. Fast, and thereby give Nature an opportunity to eliminate these "toxic waste matters," which Ehret calls "mucus." High blood pressure, migraine or other

71

types of headaches, cardiac conditions or peptic ulcers, colitis, rickets, anemia, neuritis or acidosis, epilepsy, glaucoma, urinary disturbances of the bladder, nephritis, tumors, or even sterility, to name but just a few, according to Ehret's teachings, consist of an overloaded mucus condition existing throughout the entire body, directly traceable to the one great dietetic sin—gluttonous overeating of incorrect food mixtures. Ehret's claim that 99.9 percent of all ailments actually results from the one cause—wrong food combinations and "gluttony"—remains unshaken! Forcing ourselves to eat when no appetite exists because of the prevalent and popular belief that we must eat to gain strength and vitality, can result in the temporary loss of all desire for food of any kind and, unfortunately, the results of this forced eating of—"plenty of good nourishing foods" may actually produce an entirely opposite result! We end up building disease rather than gaining vitality—and oftentimes, permanent illness is the net result! All of which teaches us that strength, vitality, and good health are by no means dependent upon the *quantity* of our food intake but rather through the actual amount of properly digested and assimilated food eaten that can be used by the body.

Fasting can start you on the road to the fulfillment of an enjoyable, pleasant, happy way of life; and the end result of following a natural method of eating and living is a longer, healthful life! These are but a few "why to fast" reasons.

When and How to Fast

Dr. Frank McCoy, in his book, *The Fast Way to Health*, recounts hundreds of cases who were greatly helped through an exclusive liquid diet consisting of nothing but fresh orange juice. The patient reported to Dr. McCoy's office daily, for periods of from 3 to 6 weeks. Besides the orange juice diet, other modalities such as massage, vibrating machines, colonic irrigations, and chiropractic adjustments were also used in the treatment to help keep the patient occupied; but Dr. McCoy gives full credit to the fast. Bernarr McFadden, the well-known Physical Culturist, received much publicity through advocating an exclusive milk diet and thousands of persons claim to have received great benefit from this diet. Both modalities—the fresh orange juice and milk diet—come under the category of what could be called a "camouflaged fast." In other words, the body is permitted to "rest" and rebuild since the one type of food only requires considerably less vitality to digest. The overworked organs are thus given an opportunity to slow down, thereby strengthening the patient's vitality. Unused morbid waste encumbrances are eliminated, and the previously overworked body can now carry on the normal digestive process. An exclusive "milk diet" can cause constipation and for this reason has proven undesirable. The fresh orange juice diet, if used by a patient heavily encumbered with concentrated poisons, could cause these concentrated poisons to be released into the bloodstream too rapidly, and in fact, it might even be conceivable, without proper supervision, this condition could end disastrously.

73

To attempt a long fast and at the same time continue to carry on our daily chores or work as usual is not entirely fair to the faster since, after all, we must not overlook the fact that during the fast we are actually on "Nature's operating table." A considerable amount of bodily vitality is consumed during the process of throwing off these age-old "poisons and toxic waste materials" and justifiably a complete rest—even to the point of remaining in bed during the entire period of the fast—is often indicated. In other words, a complete physical rest and mental relaxation should be the rule if at all possible during such strenuous "housecleansing" periods. The form of fasting known as a liquid diet, especially if the liquid consists of fresh fruit or vegetable juices or cooked vegetable broth (celery, carrots, parsley, onions, tomatoes, etc.) can be continued a month or more without overtaxing the patient's vital forces. But when fresh grapes, orange, or grapefruit juice is used exclusively, considerably more caution must be the rule since these particular juices being extremely aggressive, have a decidedly potent ability to "stir up" toxic wastes. Thrown into the blood circulation too rapidly, especially after a long total fast when the eliminated poisons are in concentrated form, the bloodstream becomes "overloaded" and normal body functioning is seriously disarranged. Dizzy spells might occur, followed by severe diarrhea and vomiting—and while this could be only temporary, it should require careful observation and attention. In case this physical reaction persists, it is advisable, and imperative to discontinue the fast immediately, and a diet of cooked vegetables containing much roughage, such as celery, carrots, cabbage, squash, spinach, beets, sauerkraut, etc., or even meats (particularly if the patient has been a one-sided meat eater) temporarily, at least until the body functioning returns to normal and all symptoms of dizziness have completely disappeared. When cooked or baked, all types of fruits and vegetables, including the fresh-frozen fruits and vegetables, are much less "aggressive" as far as their eliminating ability is concerned. Now you may appreciate why it is so necessary that you take into consideration the amount of existing waste and "poisonous" toxic matters in your body before undertaking a long fast. Even the innocent appearing "soothing syrups" given to infants contain some form of "narcotics" in minute dosage—hence, the extreme importance of having complete knowledge before suggesting a long fast is so essential in more ways than one.

We need only to look to the animal world to learn the importance that wise Mother Nature places in fasting. All sick, seriously ill, or wounded animals immediately discontinue eating food and go on a total fast in a secluded place where they can relax from all activity until they have completely regained their health and vigor. This could require a period of time as long as a week or even a month, but their patience is always rewarded with success. Complete fasting without food or water of a number of animals during their long winter hibernation is a well-known phenomenon, and it is even customary for many animals to fast during the "nursing period," remaining with their young until weaned. Fasting must be recognized as a natural and safe method of care of the sick body, a method by which the person is enabled to overcome illness through eliminating, almost miraculously, the cause of the ailment, and yet it can be said there is nothing "miraculous" about it!

Whether we fast to restore health, gain or lose weight, or merely to retain our present bodily vigor, we soon recognize that fasting is a vital factor through which we may increase our vitality and personal well-being, both mentally and physically. Besides readily overcoming such minor discomforts as the common cold or indigestion, fasting undoubtedly adds to your life span! The digestive process uses up precious vitality—contrariwise, fasting has been known to actually rebuild vital forces, and the conclusion must become self-evident that fasting prolongs life itself! It is necessary, therefore, that we repeat over and over again the importance of entering upon a fast intelligently, confident in the final outcome, with complete understanding and knowledge, and we specifically refer to the longer fasts. It is essential, for example, that the faster knows the difference between "false" and "real" appetite. Hunger pains caused through "false appetite" can generate rather severe pains in the stomach region, together with various emotional disturbances and a corresponding feeling of weakness. Since the eating of food will at this period immediately cause stoppage of the distress symptoms, it is only natural for the faster to surmise that lack of food was the cause and eating, the remedy, whereas the opposite might be true.

Our established life-long habit of eating "by the clock" has firmly affixed in our minds the desirability of eating at that precise time. The fact of the matter is that true hunger can only take place when a real need for food exists! The individual who is always hungry is, in fact, "pathologically unwell." Surely, no need for food exists when hunger is lacking. Never force yourself to eat unless you are *truly* hungry and a keen relish for food exists. Otherwise, you merely add work to an already "overworked" digestive tract. All excess food becomes a burden and this, of course, is especially true in case of illness. Overeating or forced feeding retards recovery by requiring the body to use its precious vitality in the elimination of this unneeded food. Often this so-called "good nourishing" diet is actually to blame for the patient's loss of weight and lessened vitality! Even in the healthy body, when overeating or gluttony is indulged in, it can cause vomiting and diarrhea, for the healthy organ rejects all excess food. Contrariwise, when the quantity of food intake is decreased (lessened), bodily energy is conserved since the digestive organs have less work to do—liver, pancreas, heart, and arteries are relieved of a greater portion of their labor, all of which naturally results in an increase of the healing process! Withholding all food intake from the sick patient causes every depurating organ in the entire body to increase its eliminating activity. It starts immediately to get rid of all poisonous wastes and a cleansing of the entire tissue system begins.

Nothing equals the fast as a means of eliminating age-old, stored-up wastes from an overloaded tissue system. Nature's constant and unceasing effort, therefore, is to remove all unusable and excess waste substances from the body; and fortunately for us, this constant elimination goes on continuously and good health is the result. To be willing to settle for half health or less when real health is possible is to rob yourself of life's most precious possession. Aristotle, that great Greek philosopher, said over 2,300 years ago, "If there is one way better than another, it is the way of Nature." Much vital energy is required during this cleansing process, but paradoxical as it might seem, the faster usually gains in both strength and weight. The feverish patient already lacks the necessary vitality to digest food while suffering pain, yet "nourishing food" continues to be advised. Unfortunately, the popular idea that humans must eat every few hours in order to stay alive remains, despite the fact that it has been proven over and over again that the "sick person" actually gains in strength when food is withheld, and suffers a relapse from forced feeding! How many thousands of patients have been innocently "fed" into premature graves through ignorance of Nature's laws? No claim is herein made that fasting alone, regardless of the advanced stage of the illness, or bodily and mental condition of the patient, will produce the sure cure.

Common sense and caution must be your guide during the fast, and we can safely predict that in the majority of cases the faster will become physically stronger and more vital and mentally alert—up to the point, of course, that the individual is capable of accepting. Unfortunately, fasting, when used in far-advanced cases as a last resort or in long-standing chronic cases, especially in the elderly person of lowered vitality, cannot be expected to produce the "miracle." Terminal cases, for example, can only hope for a lessening of the discomfort of their pain. Total fasting is not indicated in these terminal cases, but worthwhile results, merely through reducing the quantity of food intake, are often experienced. An extremely limited, carefully selected diet in all cases should be carried on—and, remember, overfeeding can only result in increased suffering.

Dr. J. H. Tilden, MD conducted thousands of fasts in his Denver Sanitarium and authored many books on the subject of fasting. He wrote, "I must say in all seriousness that fasting when combined with a properly selected diet is the nearest approach to a 'cure-all' that is possible to conceive—profoundly simple and simply profound!" Without exception, all of the modern "miracle drugs," including aspirin drugs employed today to restore the sick and ailing to normal health, have been known to result in great bodily harm. It is well known and readily acknowledged that they act as a palliative and not a cure, yet often the ill effects they cause are not discovered until many years after taking, before reactions occur in the affected organ and are recognized. When the cause of illness is finally removed and the restorative process of true healing is given the opportunity to function, Nature's remarkable "rebuilding" process takes place and proceeds in an orderly manner in accordance with natural physiological law! Wounds are healed, broken bones are mended, destroyed tissues are replaced, and we can positively state that these healing processes have never been duplicated through any method or laboratory finding as yet devised by mere humans! It is true that the scientist has kept living tissue alive and growing in his laboratory, but they have never been able to reproduce living tissue, nor have they developed a human-made substitute for the natural life process through which healing is accomplished!

Nature's healing process starts instantly when the need occurs, and we must recognize the importance of aiding Nature through fasting, since we now know that the healing process increases when the body is freed from disposing of surplus food. Only a total abstinence from food makes it possible for the sick body to function thoroughly, in its own inimitable way, during the healing period. As previously mentioned, Arnold Ehret preferred the so-called "short fast" of 3 days to a week or 10 days for the average individual. It was his experience that satisfactory results could be obtained through a series of so-called "shorter" fasts, especially in cases where the patient is not under competent supervision and "on his own," so to speak. It is well for the individual to decide on how long he or she intends to carry on before initiating the fast. Let us say, for example, that the patient is of the "nervous," high-strung, or imaginative type, or they may even be skeptical of results that might occur. He or she must first of all create an enthusiastic desire to fast. If the slightest doubt of final success is permitted to enter his mind, then not more than 2 or 3 days should be the extent of the fast in this case. Hopefully, the resulting good feeling will quiet all future unnecessary fears, and the next fast can be for a longer period, even up to a full week.

The overweight individual finds it much easier to go without food. Loss of weight causes no fear, and the patient's mental attitude makes fasting almost a pleasure! A week, or perhaps 10 days, for this type of individual brings practically no discomfort whatsoever. The first day's hunger pangs perhaps are the most difficult. A mouthful of water (held for 10 or 15 minutes before expectorating) will lessen the "false appetite" craving for food, which decreases as the fast progresses. The seriously sick or severely injured individual has absolutely no desire for food, so fasting comes naturally. A safe rule to follow is to stop eating until appetite has returned, or until you feel completely well.

When to Fast (Part 2)

Nature has selected the spring of the year for the annual "housecleansing" period. The very types of the first green-leaf vegetables and fruits that Nature brings forth and amply supplies in the early spring give significant testimony to this fact. The green-leaf vegetables and herbs are proven blood purifiers, well known over the centuries, and because of their laxative qualities, they are recognized efficient "cleansers." This same description applies as well to the first fruits of the season. Cherries, for example, one of the earlier fruits to ripen, have long been recognized for their "cleansing" ability. Their enticing color appeal, plus the sweet and delicious flavor, particularly when gathered and eaten direct from the tree, will produce remarkable blood-purifying and "cleansing" results. An exclusive cherry diet for 5 or 6 days is a "camouflaged fast" well worth trying. Since the body's resistance to cold weather is lowered during the fast, it is more pleasant to fast during the warmer weather; but this is not to say that we should wait until warm weather returns before undertaking a fast, if the need for fasting exists. Postponing the fast awaiting warmer weather could prove inadvisable, for a delay might conceivably result in the ailment becoming more involved. It is very easy for the patient to remain indoors while fasting and remain comfortable during the coldest weather.

Why to Fast (Part 2)

Fasting is indicated in many instances. At the first indication of the "common cold," for example, fasting becomes a preventative measure! Start the "cleansing" (fasting) program before a more serious, chronic condition develops! Minor ailments such as headaches, biliousness, nervousness, injuries, and even excessive grief all indicate the desirability of missing a meal or two. The length of time must, of course, depend entirely on the condition of the faster. For more serious ailments, the amount of toxic waste and foreign encumbrances present in the bloodstream must be taken into consideration, and often a longer fast is indicated. Age of the faster is another important factor, since we cannot expect to overcome the effects of a lifetime of wrong living within a few short days or weeks. The chronic sufferer, therefore, must exercise patience and perseverance in his efforts to return to normal health. It is to be expected that in many instances the faster becomes discouraged, even frightened, at the actual results that the fast brings about during the early stages of the "housecleaning" period. But with complete faith and knowledge of what is actually occurring, the final results will eventually prove very worthwhile. A little "self-discipline" would provide many of us with a steady flow of energy and a wonderful sense of inner well-being that comes from a healthy body.

Where to Fast

Often times, where to fast must be given a great deal of consideration. The inevitable opposition of the well-meaning members of the "family" often proves to be the most difficult of the obstacles to overcome. Our loved ones, because of the inborn fear of starvation inculcated in all of us since early childhood, find it impossible to withhold well-intentioned warnings, and often plead tearfully with the faster to "eat something." They honestly and sincerely believe that great bodily harm, even death itself, will inevitably result from a fast of more than a few days at most! Their pleadings, when ignored, often lead to hysterical and angry efforts to force the faster to "eat some good nourishing food," and the unfortunate sick person, already weakened through illness, loses his or her original determination to "get well or else"—and succumbs to their pleadings by "eating something," which often are the very foods that should not be used! It may well be that the faster is not completely "sold" to the efficacy of the fast—in which case the faster can be more easily swayed from their original plan to continue the fast, since they lack the courage of their own convictions. Should this experience be yours, then at least eat the foods that you know are indicated for breaking the fast, as taught by Prof. Arnold Ehret, in order to accomplish the most good. It might be wise under these conditions to arrange for suitable supervision at a sanitarium or rest home specializing in fasting, particularly if the faster contemplates a longer fast of two or 3-weeks duration. Never lose sight of the fact that the faster is on "Nature's 'bloodless' operating table" and should, therefore, be made comfortable at all times through adequate nursing care, daily sponge baths, massage, colonic irrigations, with complete rest and relaxation, so that the bodily strength and comfort can be retained and even increased. To obey Nature's laws means health—to disregard, whether through ignorance or deliberately, means pain, disease, and even death. In other words, health is not merely an accident but an achievement—for the orderly working of the body functions spells HEALTH and its derangement results in disease. The warning signs of pain and discomfort signify that Nature's laws have been digressed, whether unintentionally or not! Freedom from pain, or HEALTH, means that they have been complied with. In the overwhelming majority of illness, all that Nature requires for health to be gained is a discontinuance from doing that which was the original cause of the disease—yet our natural instinct to fast, even missing a single meal, has become lost through present-day "civilization," and the increase in all human ills can be directly traced to the accepted customs of our advanced "civilization."

How Long to Fast

The exact length of the fast need not be *definitely* decided beforehand. The various physical and mental reactions that take place during the fast could understandably often cause needless alarm to both the faster and the inexperienced physician. For the first time in years, possibly for the first time in the life of the faster, a thorough cleansing of the tissue system is possible, and stored-up toxemic wastes and poisons are now being carried off as the avenues of circulation contract, permitting the existing overpressure to be rapidly relieved. Renewed vitality enables the bloodstream to discharge the dissolved mucus and toxemic waste materials now in circulation for elimination, and these "poisonous encumbrances" might cause a feeling of being "ill" to exist during this period. You will find, however, that just as soon as the "cleansing process" is completed and the wastes are eliminated, the faster feels stronger than ever before! Ehret often remarked about his fasting patients actually feeling stronger on the third week of the fast than they did during the first week! The unobstructed blood circulation can now produce increased vitality—further proof that Nature heals through fasting. It is this elimination of waste, poisonous materials with which the tissues and intestinal tract have been "clogged up" for years and now finally removed, that make it possible for normal bodily function to once again take place. It is Nature alone, in the final analysis, through fasting and the resulting elimination of waste materials through the various depurating organs, i.e., the skin, kidneys, lungs, bowels, as well as our eyes, ears, and nose that aid the true healing process to take place. "The mills of the Gods grind slowly, yet they grind exceedingly fine!"

In the final summation, we cannot emphasize too strongly the fact that what we know as disease is in reality a "process of purification"—a special effort as it were, on the part of the abused, sick organism to throw off the abnormal quantities of latent poisonous-waste materials. Our perverted dietetic habits, the result of false teachings since childhood, are the origin. We attempt to "stop" the pain through unnatural means rather than recognize pain as Nature's warning signal of a local symptom of a general disorder. The majority of persons, never having experienced the feeling of real health and vitality, are not cognizant of what they are missing. They little suspect that humankind's greatest enemies—ignorance, selfishness, greed, and gluttony, the cause of all his or her physical and mental woes exist within himself! Discontinue careless and indulgent overeating! Comply with Nature's unchangeable laws for safe guidance in your search for health! Fasting gives the body an opportunity to correct these faults of improper dieting—and incompatible food combinations. To enjoy this more abundant, healthier life is within your reach. The sooner you make the decision to start, the better off you surely will be. Why not grasp this opportunity and let us help you attain your desired goal of a longer, happier, healthier, more vigorous life.

Become a disciple of health and prove to yourself that strict self-discipline brings worthwhile results. Then, through precept and example, hold high the torch of knowledge and enlightenment to your fellow humans who, while teetering on the very brink of physical and mental collapse, find themselves still unable to grasp these simple truths or understand the cause of their suffering. Make them anxious to travel the broad road to health leading to a completely new—wonderful, joyous—life of physical, spiritual, and mental regeneration.

- FINIS -

SECTION III

ROADS TO HEALTH AND HAPPINESS

PART I

Your Road to Regeneration:

Building Bodily Strength and Efficiency

By Arnold Ehret

It was during my early thirties that I first became severely sick with Bright's disease and on the very verge of the grave. Even after being told by orthodox medical physicians that my illness was incurable, I fought my way up to an unshaken health that still remains today—a health far better than in the best years of my youth, when I did my military service. I found more or less temporary relief through different methods of Nature-cure and drugless healing as practiced at that time, but it became necessary for me to return to nature's infallible remedies—the only methods that can truly overcome disease, and they are fasting and an exclusive fruit diet!

Neither of these unfailing, healing factors were given practically any consideration nor credit for their potential healing abilities by any of the various healing arts of that time. In fact, even today, acknowledgment still continues to be sorely lacking—by both medical science and the average lay person who might be interested in their own health regime, but who continues to remain sublimely ignorant. It took years of study, testing, and self-experimentation, which often bordered upon the dangerous, before I finally came upon the truth. And the TRUTH is this! No matter what you may be suffering from, regardless of how feverish, weak, or desperately ill you may feel, NATURE WANTS TO SAVE YOU! Disease is merely Nature's effort to start performing the process of healing—the elimination of wastes and disease matters that clog up your tissue system. Listen to the instinctive advice of Nature unfailingly given to both humans and animals: "Give me a chance to eliminate; to repair your bodily mechanism!" "Take time to be "sick" for a few days or even weeks, and I will help you!" "Remain still, quiet, rest, sleep, and DON'T EAT!"

When you obstruct Nature's good intentions through the use of human-made synthetic drugs, or continue eating more and more of the disease-producing foods, or if the quantities of waste, mucus, and poisons in your body are too much and too old, then Nature cannot help and you must die just as animals do who fail to recuperate through fasting alone. In fact, it is through this very method that Nature wipes out the weak, the degenerated ones who violated nature's laws of living, whether deliberately or innocently through ignorance. The natural tendency of evolution seeks as a goal not quantity but quality! It is truly indicative of how far humans have degenerated through wrong living, especially through wrong eating.

The selection and preparation of his or her various foods become immensely important factors of life when one recognizes that a large percentage of all humankind living today could not endure a long fast! You can learn more about these surprising facts in my book, the *MUCUSLESS DIET HEALING SYSTEM*. Without a corrective diet, a perfect health CANNOT be attained through modern miracle drugs or any form of accepted remedies or through mechanical treatments. A supreme, absolute, Paradisiacal health—the way of infallible healing—must be achieved through, and is ruled by, the laws of diet. Humans, like every living plant and organism, mature and owe their existence to food. Human health and disease of every description directly result from food intake. Their state of mind may be a contributing factor, but the fall of humankind in the final analysis is "sin of diet." The real physiological cause of all evils, especially the physical ailments of humankind, can be traced directly to the present-day accepted diet of civilization. Having allowed your body to degenerate through overeating wrong, disease-producing food, prayer alone will prove unavailing without a physical effort being made to correct your wrong living habits.

Humankind's salvation and their return to the ideal prototype of the "perfect" normal being will require a complete healing from the "sins of the diet of civilization" as practiced today. Disease is internal uncleanliness acquired over all ages by wrong foods. My revelation of diseases and their healing through corrective diet is based on proof and backed by experience and experiments conducted on my own body as well as thousands of patients at my Sanitarium in Switzerland during a period of over 15 years. All methods of natural treatments are indeed more or less cleansing, healing, and even more or less rejuvenating, but fail to completely overcome the SOURCE, which is the direct cause of the "clogging-up" condition. A well-selected "cleansing" diet consisting of fresh fruits and green-leaf vegetables makes it a distinct pleasure rather than a "painful" experience. The different kinds of food making many variations possible, the prescribed rest and relaxation are all indicated in each individual case, and therefore must be especially selected to meet the varying situations. For example, a careful determination of the quantity of waste and poisons in the daily elimination of mucus now being dissolved and carried off by the bloodstream should be recognized.

The coated tongue and the sample specimen of urine, the putrid fecal matter, are all telltale stories. The vital efficiency of the patient should not be obstructed, and therefore a "slowing-down" of the aggressive effect of elimination is advisable. The more time allowed for the body to throw off the stored up poisons, the less vitality will be required to do the work and the more certain of success in the treatment! For example: where the case history shows that "drugs" have been used over a long period of time, it becomes extremely advisable to "slow-down" the aggressive effect of elimination through the use of cooked foods—especially vegetables containing roughage, such as found in beets, beet tops, spinach, celery, etc. If the "ailment" is at all remediable, Nature heals not only the disease but also the whole person! It may require as long as 1 to 3 years of systematically continued natural-cleansing diets and fasting for the average "sick" person before the body is cleansed of "foreign matters." Assuring results will of course be noticed within the first few weeks. You may then see how the body is constantly eliminating waste from the urinary canal, the colon, the eyes, ears, nose, and throat—from every pore of the skin over the entire surface of the body! You will observe how both "wet" and "dried" mucus (dandruff, scaly formations in the nose, wax in the ear drums, for instance) is being continuously expelled. You will then readily agree with me when I state that all diseases of humankind, both mental and physical—ever since the beginning of our civilization—have the same foundational cause, whatever the symptoms may be! It is without a single exception one. and the same universal condition—a "one-ness" of all disease—and that is: waste, foreign matter, excess mucus, and their related poisons, i.e., stench (offensive odor) or "invisible waste."

Everyone, no matter to what extent they may claim to enjoy "good health," has a latent sickness! A severe "shock," such as the so-called "cold" or "influenza," starts the elimination throughout the entire body. This attempted "housecleaning" by Mother Nature should not be interfered with by either continued eating or the use of drug suppressants. Nature should be permitted to eliminate this excess waste, often stored in the body since early childhood! Interference often results in producing "acute" and "chronic" diseases. It goes without saying that the process of elimination is not a pleasant experience, but how self-satisfying it is to know positively that you have averted a more severe stage of the illness that a postponement would have eventually made necessary. The human's mastery of disease will bring humanity closer to perfection of the human body. If you hope to achieve good health, freedom from pain and all illness, and the full enjoyment of a paradisiacal existence, it can be obtained through proper observance of Nature's laws pertaining to the creation of humans themselves.

The truth of my statements are self-evident—and humankind will continue to go on and on, suffering never-ending aches and pains—until the truth shall set them free. No one needs to live with disease—and freedom from disease has now become a reality. My *Mucusless Diet Healing System* has brought to all who would listen and heed all of the information needed to banish illness and suffering from disease. Cleansing is basic for the correction and elimination of all disorders from which humans suffer, caused through the accumulation of poisons and congestion throughout the entire body. Unusable and accumulated waste stored in the tissues cause degeneration and decay. When we stop feeding and cleanse our system, we allow the body to return to normalcy. "Magic cures," "witchcraft," or "miracle drugs" cannot possibly eliminate the cause of any disease. The "cleansing diet" is at the same time a "body-building" diet—leaving the body free from the accumulation of toxic waste, brought about through the eating of "mucus-forming" foods. Skin disorders and other conditions such as, boils, abscesses, and carbuncles—Nature's untiring effort to eliminate excess waste and poisons—will disappear quickly from the body. Correct foods (fruits and green-leaf vegetables) permit Nature to build a strong, healthy body; wrong foods produce a diseased body. We can eliminate all suffering, ailments, and disease through the physiological operations of diet. As the goal of the infallible true food of humans, you will find in Genesis 1:29 a biological law of eating. Foods manufactured and prepared by humans only cause disease, troubles, and sickness, and are therefore "wrong foods." Right foods—fresh fruits and green-leaf vegetables—are healthy, divine foods, healing and disease-free; paradisiacal living! Believing, knowing, having complete faith in these truthful facts and their scientific application, is the infallible principles of all healing, the REAL knowledge that must eventually result in the physiological salvation of humankind. Humans today consume too much food—not too little! We must realize the limitations of the human digestive system.

I now have successfully solved the problem through a scientifically correct system, and I can unequivocally state the following truth: "DISEASE is Nature's effort to rid the body of 'disease matters' and eliminate waste from the system."

The deeper causes of internal uncleanliness and its resulting constipation can be definitely corrected and overcome through my teachings, not merely relieved! This has proven to be the one sane, useable, and scientific road to regeneration. The simplicity and naturalness of these methods cannot help but appeal to the intelligent lay person interested in self-betterment—physical, mental, and spiritual.

You now hold in your hands a scientific source of diet information, a cleansing diet nature intended for the use of humans, a diet that can rid your system of disease-causing, poisonous filth— truly the discovery of the "Road to Health."

- FINIS -

PART II

My Road to Health

By Teresa Mitchell

Preface

I have been an Ehret devotee for the past 25 years and I shall remain so until the end of my days. My greatest desire is to share with others the wonderful results I have gained, both in physical and mental health.

The experiences outlined in the following article, "My Road To Health," are of course all true. Were I to continue rewriting these experiences for the next 10 years, the wording and phrasing might be improved, but the truth must always remain the same. I shall always consider my experiences with the Ehret diet the greatest accomplishment of my entire life!

When I think of the benefits that could accrue to the human race were we to renounce the foods of present-day civilization and return to a diet of natural, unadulterated foods such as taught by Prof. Ehret, my heart becomes heavy and I find it almost more than I can bear. The problem, therefore, is how to convince others of these truths. I can only hope that I have been the means of pointing the way even in some small degree.

It is the average person that I am anxious to reach, so that they may be led ever so gently on to the right path in matters of diet. I consider the *Mucusless Diet Healing System* so great a benefaction to humankind that I feel it should have all the publicity possible, not for monetary gain, but for more noble and humanitarian reasons and the love of our fellow humans.

Health is within everyone's grasp—all we need do is reach for it. Perhaps it will be difficult in the beginning—it might even take considerably longer than we would like—but in the end, our efforts will surely be crowned with the energy that radiates from a healthy body and which ultimately brings success and happiness.

-Teresa Mitchell

My Road to Health

It all started many years ago in the war-torn country of Hungary. The many privations, frustrating experiences, and abuses our family had been subjected to during the troubled times of the first World War had undoubtedly served to develop an intense desire on my part to overcome the conditions into which I, together with others of my class, had been tossed. When World War I finally ended, mother and I were most fortunate in being presented with an opportunity to immigrate to this greatest of all countries, the United States of America. We gratefully embraced the chance and left for the land of our dreams just as fast as it was legally possible for us to do. America proved to be unbelievably wonderful—far beyond my most imaginative dreams.

Adjusting ourselves to American ways of living, but more especially adapting ourselves to American eating habits, was not particularly easy. The change from the meager rations of our wartime diet to the abundance of the American diet soon proved my physical undoing. During the war period, our diet in Hungary was practically meatless and sugarless. Now in America, I could have as much meat, pastries, sugar, and dairy products that I wanted—just the kind of food I had been craving—without any restriction on quantities. This was America, the land of plenty—truly a land of milk and honey. I soon found my health declining. Continued illness led to consultations with doctors who informed me that possibly the drastic change in food could be responsible. Fortunately for me, through the help of new-found friends, I learned of the wonderful, free public libraries where many books on diet could be found. I avidly read most of them, for they interested me greatly, particularly those dealing with vegetarian diets. Gradually, I began to apply many of the diet suggestions to my own eating habits. The results proved extremely gratifying, for unwittingly I had returned to my previous vegetarian diet. The first proof of good results was when I found that I no longer needed reading glasses, after having worn them for the previous 3 years. I joined a hiking club and learned to enjoy the great outdoors climbing mountains and spending the day close to Nature's secrets. Our hike leader taught us common-sense breathing exercises during the frequent but short rest periods while we were on our hikes. At last, I felt that I had discovered the right way for me to live.

95

Surely now I would be most happy to live this way the remainder of my life. And then, most fortunately for me, I learned about a book called the *Mucusless Diet Healing System* written by Prof. Arnold Ehret. I still treasure my copy of this marvelous book, whose dog-eared pages I still read and reread (even after 27 years) and continue to find wonderful. This book was the real stepping stone to my Shangri-La of Health. This Shangri-La was not a place cloistered by tall mountains, reached only after grueling effort and hardship by only a few determined and courageous souls. No, on the contrary, my Shangri-La is readily accessible to everyone wanting to enter through its doors.

I soon learned that all I had heretofore read about health and diet was only partly right. But now, with my new knowledge plus courage, faith, and backbone, perfect health was actually within my grasp and could be achieved through the understandable teachings contained in this remarkable book. Almost immediately, I felt the author's sincerity and accepted every word of his teachings. Instinctively, I knew that this time I was on the right track. After many months of following the "Transition Diet" as taught by Ehret, the cleansing I achieved startled me. Yes, the effectiveness of the diet was unquestionable. A miracle in healing had taken place right under my very eyes. For instance, a goiter that had already become annoyingly obvious on my neck completely disappeared! I could not believe it possible to feel any better than I now felt. Various minor symptoms, almost too numerous to mention, likewise disappeared.

Two years had passed since I first began the transition diet, and by then, I truly relished all of the foods that were allowed me. I earnestly followed the exercises given in the book, as well as developing some of my own. A fine breathing exercise, which I discovered, helped me overcome the weakness that often accompanies a drastic diet change. The time was now approaching when the final great step for complete healing, as taught by Prof, Ehret, should be taken. The decision was not easy. I began questioning myself, "Do I dare take it?" "Why go further since I really feel fine now." "I must be physically all right for it has been a long time since I have had even a 'simple' cold." As I kept arguing with myself, strange thoughts as well as doubts came into my mind. "Suppose the author was wrong—it is barely possible that they might be mistaken in his conclusions." While Ehret taught "human's food is fruits and green-leaf vegetables," how could anyone possibly exist on such a monotonous diet? "Is my willpower strong enough?"

I began to discuss Prof. Ehret's teachings with others who, like me, were interested in regaining health through diet. Some had made an attempt, but not one among them went all the way through with the diet. "It takes too much willpower," I was told by some, while others said, "You'll dry up," or "Your bones will become brittle through lack of calcium." "Modern civilization makes it impossible." Others, apparently more kindly, admonished, "Why do it—is it not enough that you are healthy now?" "You will be all alone in your belief—no one will understand you." How I longed to take my problems directly to Prof. Ehret, but at the very pinnacle of success that he had unfortunately met with a fatal accident. After a long and careful review of the "pros and cons," I came to the decision that my life was my own and I would do with it as I saw fit. I seemed to realize that until I had thoroughly tried Ehret's teachings, I could know no real feeling of success. All fear left as soon as my decision was made and I decided to confide in no one. My goal was to "taste of Paradise," as Ehret had promised. This experimenting with restricted diets had now been going on for a period of years and ironically enough, during the entire period the only jobs available to me were in restaurants—either cashier, food checker, or waitress.

My decision made, I started out early one morning with determination in my heart. I halfway expected everything and everyone to be different—but upon my arrival at work, everyone and everything was the same as always—the tantalizing smells of frying bacon and "ham and eggs," the urn full of steaming coffee, and the trays heavily laden with food. The few early-morning, sleepy-eyed women, the men patrons in grimy coats and their work-stained overalls—all were the same as before. As a matter of fact, only one thing was actually different—and that was my mental attitude, which no one seemed to notice—not immediately, or for a while at least, that is to say.

A Difficult First Week

It was no easy matter to live up to this decision of remaining on a strict fruit diet until complete healing of my body was accomplished.

Over and over again, I had to remind myself of the blessings I had hoped to gain, and only by holding a mental picture of success in front of me more times than I care to admit, the first week finally passed. I daresay this first week was the hardest part of the entire venture. Having no precedent to go by as to the right amount of fruit that I should eat at one meal, I did a little experimenting. Fortunately, watermelons were in season and I soon found them to be more filling than most other fruits. Co-workers and friends began to notice the monotony of my meals, and I found it difficult to keep my secret. Finally, I decided to confide in the manager, and he understandably told others about it. From then on, I was a "freak" among the employees. but fortunately, it did not bother me too much.

My previous years on vegetarian diets proved advantageous, having conditioned me, more or less, for an exclusive fruitarian diet; yet, it is true, I lost considerable weight. The vegetarian diet had accomplished a lot of good results in the elimination of toxic encumbrances and waste matter, and the toxin-producing meat and dairy products had no part in my diet for the past number of years. However, frequent expectoration continued for a long time while on the fruit regime, and I also noticed considerable elimination of stringy mucus accompanying my stool. Yet there were many indications of general improvement in my health, which gave me increased determination to go on with my experiment.

The skin on my face, which had seemed to sag after the first 10 days or 2 weeks, became firm and smooth again after a period of a month's time. My eyes became clear and bright and a new feeling of exhilaration came over me. This was something I had seldom experienced, if at all. I decided I must be making progress.

The grape season was now on hand and I found all varieties of grapes to be a satisfying food. While Muscat grapes seemed to be the most pleasing and satisfying to me, I enjoyed any kind of grapes. I soon discovered that it required only about an hour for fruits to digest, and I therefore ate whenever I would feel the gnawing pangs of hunger. But—and this is extremely important—I learned that even fruits have a harmful reaction if one overeats of them! Nature has a very subtle way of letting us know when we have eaten enough.

A Workable Diet

This new habit of eating whenever I felt hunger pangs proved difficult to manage during working hours. When I thought that no one was looking, I would sneak a bite from an apple or other fruit that I had hidden near the cash register. The manager soon put an end to this surreptitious eating, but he kindly suggested that I help myself to whatever fruit might be in the refrigerator. Needless to say, this made life much easier. What was most amazing to me was that I had not become weakened through this strict fruit diet. While I had been forewarned that I might even become bedfast for a time, the "weakness" I had been led to expect failed to materialize. I did not miss one single day from my work.

I love to sing, and on frequent occasions I have been told that I have a fairly good voice, so during the previous 2 years I had been taking vocal lessons. After 3 months on this rigid diet, my teacher remarked about a decided change that was taking place in the quality of my voice, as well as decided changes in my general appearance and personality. It seemed that I had more breath and better control, and that my voice had more resonance—in fact, had become much clearer. I was thrilled with this progress but still hesitated about revealing my diet to my teacher for I enjoyed the moral strength that keeping this secret seemed to give me.

Even after 6 months of my exclusive fruit diet, I still had not reached the point where, according to Prof. Ehret's teachings, all obstacles would be swept aside. Living in a rooming house completely alone, with Mother, my only living relative in this country, thousands of miles away (she had remained in Ohio when I came to California), I was finding it a difficult fight. Mother and I corresponded regularly, yet I never revealed my diet to her for fear of being discouraged by her. Encouragement was what I most needed at this point of the experiment. Loneliness was probably the most difficult of all the obstacles I had to battle. I tried to keep my mind occupied through reading and planning the things I would like to do after reaching my goal with the diet. Despite the many friends I made with almost everyone with whom I came in contact, that strange loneliness still persisted. With the arrival of Fall came apple time. I fondly recall the delicious Jonathan apples that helped to vary my diet. A large-sized Jonathan made a complete meal in itself.

By this time, I had been living on the fruitarian diet for about 9 months, and many encouraging and wonderful things had taken place. For at least the past 2 months, I had felt like a newborn babe. How I wanted to shout this message from the housetops. "This must be the way God intended humans to live. Why won't people accept these teachings—or at least try for themselves, so that they might enjoy the truth." In my enthusiasm, I dreamed of having a whole colony of people living this Paradisiacal life. To my young mind, this was the answer to all of the ills of humanity and loneliness as well.

My skin texture became like that of a baby. The natural red of my lips no longer made the use of lipstick necessary. My eyes were clear and bright at all times. In fact, my entire being was gradually taking on a complete change. Yes, even my disposition changed for the better and a natural display of quick temper had given way to a quiet philosophic attitude toward all people and their daily problems. Fears, with which I was formerly plagued, were gradually disappearing. My thinking had changed completely. People constantly remarked about the natural and spontaneous smile that lighted my face. There was no effort needed to produce it. This wonderful feeling of exhilaration became part of my life. It was my first conscious thought upon awakening every morning.

The First Cleansing

Then the first great event happened. One night, after a supper of grapes, I was awakened by a sensation of fullness in my throat. I had no particular feeling of nausea or pain, but upon reaching the bathroom, I threw up large quantities of a sticky, clear substance. After this ordeal was over, I felt a new sense of well-being come over me. New strength and power seemed to fill my whole being. I thought this must be the great final cleansing that Prof. Ehret taught us to expect. However, it was only a forerunner of two more similar experiences before the long-expected day arrived.

During this period of cleansing and elimination, many interesting things took place—in fact, too many to enumerate here. One of the most outstanding facts, I think, was the complete absence of fatigue. My work required that I remain constantly on my feet for 8 hours, and yet after a full day's work I felt just as fresh as though I had not worked at all. The only way I knew that rest was required by my body was a feeling of drowsiness. Upon arriving home, I usually took a short nap, after which I was ready for my vocal studies at the studio. My rest at night was complete and undisturbed, for I seldom dreamed. Upon awakening, there was that indescribable clear-headedness which must be experienced in order to be understood and appreciated. No stimulants, such as coffee or tea, were needed to get me in good humor for the day's work. Thinking was becoming increasingly easier and I was actually becoming witty. In fact, I had never been aware of this gift in my adopted English language. I felt proud of my ability to give back a quick answer, as well as a ready comeback to "small" talk. My powers of concentration had become more acute. In fact, neither noises nor confusion could distract my thinking. My shyness and reticence were being replaced by poise.

Many daily temptations had to be overcome, such as when an urgent desire for foods that I knew to be harmful presented itself. I learned through repetition that the sooner I told myself, "NO." the easier it became to say "NO" the next time. A realization soon came to me that keeping my mind occupied with other things, instead of permitting thoughts of food to form, helped increase my willpower.

My residence was close to the restaurant, so that I could walk to and from work. There was one exceptionally steep hill to climb, which would invariably cause me to puff and pant. One afternoon on my way home, I felt inspired to create a poem. As the sentences took form, I became deeply engrossed in thought—when suddenly I noticed I had climbed more than halfway up the hill, yet I had felt no exertion whatever. It was as though I had been walking on level ground, and I could scarcely believe what was happening. I concluded that I must have been so engrossed in the poem that I forgot about my body. This, then, was an opportune time to make a test, so I decided to return to the bottom of the hill and walk up again, this time giving no thought to the poem. What I discovered was unbelievable. I felt as though my body had no weight at all. Here was I, ascending this steep incline, which in all probability is at least 60 percent grade, without the slightest feeling of fatigue whatsoever. I am sure that I could have easily run all the way up, and I would have tried it too, except I feared I would cause consternation among the

101

puffing and panting pedestrians. It was difficult for me to restrain myself from stopping my fellow pedestrians and telling them all about it. "I must be at the very gates of Shangri La," I thought to myself, "To think that diet could do all this."

After my enthusiasm calmed down a bit, and after considerable thought, I decided to tell certain people whom I believed might understand. While some marveled at my willpower, others simply refused to believe my story, and still others felt that while it might be a good thing for me, it surely would not be the right procedure for them to follow. It was discouraging to have people say, "You are young—it is your youth." "Yes," I answered, "I am young. Just how young do you think I am?" "Well, you can't be more than 16." When I gave my age as 26, they were incredulous.

Within myself, I knew all was well and I continued eating my fruit meals. Other seemingly unexplainable experiences followed. My feeling of well-being was boundless—I knew I was now completely restored to perfect health—I had arrived at my long hoped-for goal. No aches and pains, no physical discomfort of any kind, no headaches, no colds. This might be a good time to mention another of the "experiences" that were occurring to me. My menstrual periods only occurred at 6-month intervals, and when they did come, I felt no nervous reaction or mental depression and absolutely no pain whatsoever. Their duration was very short.

Words seem inadequate to describe the perfect state of well-being I was now privileged to experience. Sound in body, health, and mind, I considered myself fortunate indeed. The thrill of being alive was so intense that I felt this great thrill must be shared with others, for to keep it a secret was surely a sin. No doubt about it, I was an entirely different person, living in a private Paradise all my own, wonderful beyond description—calm, serene, and the few talents with which God had endowed me greatly improved.

It was my looks, my general appearance, which most certainly showed the greatest improvement. Despite a loss of twenty-five pounds, I by no means looked "skinny." I was slender in body, yes, but my face was gently rounded and my skin was like that of a baby. I was bubbling over with happiness at all times, and a glow of radiance seemed to emanate from me, since people continually remarked about it. Complete calmness and a feeling of confidence, like the confidence a small child must feel sitting in the lap of his or her mother, safe from outside harm, invaded me. Perhaps I had better describe it as sitting in the lap of God, with a small inner voice reassuring me that I was at last free from all disease. So long as my bloodstream remained clean and pure, and my tissues were no longer clogged with the encumbrances of foreign waste matter, no outside germs could attack and harm my physical body. This was a staggering realization, to say the least, and I wanted to make the most of it.

In discussing my experiences with others, I was not too surprised to learn that they had tried to live on the Ehret diet but failed. Either through lack of faith or lack of willpower, possibly both, they quit too soon. They had missed the great realization, so important to one's future life. Those who failed probably brand the Ehret teachings as unsound, but so far as I am concerned, everything taught by the author in his *Mucusless Diet Healing System* is true. I have personally proven that every statement contained in Prof. Ehret's book is based on a solid foundation of undeniable truth. This then, is the kind of health the average person cannot even conceive of, with every organ and cell of the body completely free and able to function as God intended it should, without obstructions of any kind. Probably Prof. Ehret was the only man in recent history to achieve this perfect health.

I have proven to my complete satisfaction the human body does not need the scientifically prepared foods and complicated diets that present-day civilization has come to accept as absolutely essential for health. I now know that the human body, after it has been cleansed of all the dross refuse (waste encumbrances that our modern diet leaves in every cell and in every drop of the bloodstream), can exist on fruits alone, and be marvelously healthy. And I have found that even the youngest infant must first go through a diet of cleansing before they can be fed on this "diet of Paradise," as the author called it.

Prof. Ehret's *Mucusless Diet* truly possesses the potentialities of saving this mixed-up world of ours with a rebirth of spirituality difficult to conceive even in the twentieth century. All of the five senses became keener: clearer vision, brighter colors, sounds, even whispers became distinctly audible, and re-awakened taste buds made flavors tastier and scents keener. Small wonder I still inwardly weep when I think of the misery, pain, fear, plus all of the other trials and tribulations, which make living so difficult. I became heartsick when I watched people carrying trays laden with at least five times as much food as the capacity of their stomach. Their poor, overworked organs lacked sufficient vitality to dispose of this excess quantity of waste. Small wonder they were continually "sick"—small wonder they were always tired and worn out.

Today, after a span of 27 years, my faith in the efficacy of Ehret's *Mucusless Diet Healing System* is stronger than it ever was during my younger days of experimenting. At the age of 53, I am proudly beginning to admit my age. For years, I had fibbed about it, especially to my employers. Now, my neighbors and co-workers look at me with great surprise. I am told that I should never admit to being more than 36 or 37 at the most. My skin (I must admit, at the risk of seeming to brag) still has the unwrinkled smoothness of a much younger woman. My hair is in excellent condition. I have retained a youthful, streamlined figure. My voice, which I use a great deal as a soloist, is still young and vibrant. I keep up an extensive vocal repertoire. I still enjoy the zest, capacity, and strength for work. I do all my own housework and carry on a 7- or 8-hour job outside my home. I take care of such duties as two growing sons and a husband. In my spare time, I try my hand at writing. I am completely without aches or pains of any kind, although I have been going through the difficult period of menopause. However, the generally accepted symptoms that plague the average woman during this period of life have had very slight effects on me. I have not had "shots," pills, or tonics—in fact, I have had no need to even seek the advice of a physician. My medicine cabinet is still free of pills, physics, or tonics, and I do not use creams and beauty preparations.

Needless to say, I do not wander off the straight and narrow path as laid down by Prof. Ehret in his wonderful book, which I am sure does not need my testimonial, for it has stood on its own merits for many years. Over a hundred thousand persons have already read the book and many must believe its teachings just as I do. But, may I emphasize just one point, and it is this: Whoever desires to become a disciple of Ehret's teachings should himself attain a complete healing.

Then, and then only, is he or she competent to teach the principles of "How to Control One's Health" through fasting and diet, without fear of unknown disease that might be lurking in the tissues and bloodstream of the body.

Only this can give the soul and mind of humans the freedom Nature intended us to possess.

Build Your Own Road to Health

By Teresa Mitchell

Everyone can create their own perfect health, regardless of age or condition. This might seem like a bold statement to make, but I assure you it is true. If you are willing to make the effort, to learn to have faith, and to teach yourself perseverance, *you can have perfect health*.

Rejuvenation is within your reach: a life full of action, accomplishment, and most certainly, full of the joy of living; a sane and well-balanced life that affords no time for frustrations or neuroses.

All through the history of humankind, old age has been pictured as the burdensome years, the years of decline, of senility—and ailments. But this no longer has to be so. Actually, the most rewarding and productive period of your life should be during these advanced years. This time of maturity should be spent doing the type of work requiring the experience that only a mature mind possesses. By this time, too, a certain amount of economic stability has been established. But, alas, in our present so-called civilized condition, with but few exceptions, we are too senile and too ill to enjoy fully this wonderful freedom and security. Too many of us are relegated to park benches, hoping to relieve our aching bones and throbbing joints by basking in the sunshine.

The crippling diseases of old age need never occur nor should degenerative diseases be taken for granted at any age. But unfortunately, humans continually try unnatural methods to heal themselves and in that lay their downfall.

Fortunately, Arnold Ehret, in his *Mucusless Diet Healing System*, teaches methods in complete harmony with natural laws—methods that he followed to heal himself completely. He points out that Nature's laws are immutable. Humans must first learn to subjugate themselves and then fully cooperate with the laws if they would enjoy physical and mental harmony.

Anyone seriously contemplating the truly inspiring journey to perfect health through the pages of Ehret's *Mucusless Diet Healing System* must realize that it requires careful study and intelligent judgment. The lessons contained in the book must be studied thoroughly and many times over so that the thoughts of this great health teacher become familiar. There are several very important points you must remember.

If you are suffering from an ailment pronounced "incurable," you cannot possibly expect the same immediate results as someone suffering from a minor ailment. Age, too, is necessarily an important factor. The same reaction cannot be expected by a person in their seventies as an individual in the thirties, twenties, or younger.

You must condition yourself in both body and mind to achieve the best results. For example, the three-time-a-day meat eaters should not suddenly deprive themselves of all meat products. This would prove a tremendous shock physically as well as mentally. It would be much wiser for you to cut down on food portions over a period of months and then gradually eliminate one meat meal (preferably breakfast). After a few months, you can eliminate the lunch meat dish and then you can leave off meat at dinner. Substitute a cooked vegetable plate that you really enjoy in place of the meat dish. This tapering-off system can be just as successfully applied in eliminating coffee, tea, carbohydrates, eggs, dairy products, etc.

A tapering-off system serves many purposes. First of all, it begins the disciplining of the mind that is so essential to success in this undertaking. Secondly, it begins the gradual elimination of the acids and pus in the system. Thirdly, it reduces the size of the stomach, if the suggestion not to overeat is followed.

From Wrong to Right

The transition diet set forth in the book is just what its name implies: a transition from a previous wrong way of eating to the correct, new way. The most important thing accomplished through this new regimen is the elimination of accumulated wastes with its resultant healing. First, the tottering structure is slowly and gradually torn down and the debris removed to make room for the new and modern structure.

Many students believe it is necessary to eat larger portions of fruits and vegetables when on the transition diet, since it does not have the heavier consistency of today's conventional diet. But this is not so. You actually need less fruits and vegetables, since they contain more food value. You will be surprised at the small amount of food your body really needs to nourish itself. If you eat more food than you need, this surplus food must be eliminated, and so your organs of elimination may be overworked. Gas may form if too much fruit is eaten at one time, and fruit mixed with starches tends to form gas.

It would be wise for you to eat slowly and *you should never eat unless hungry*. Nature has a very definite signal by which she lets us know when the meal is over. You must learn to heed this signal. Often acid pangs are mistakenly thought to be hunger pangs. (There is a similarity.) These false hunger pangs will disappear as the surplus acids are eliminated. Acid pangs come and go while hunger pangs persist.

Some people complain about leaving the table unsatisfied after an all-fruit meal. This is understandable, for back of all of us is a lifetime of wrong habits that require time to change. You must actually make a conscious effort to change your ideas on food and nutrition. One habit that must be broken is the one of expecting a "stuffy" or "full" feeling at the end of a meal. Relish the new kind of food in your thoughts, and I am sure you will soon like it well enough to look forward to your next meal.

109

You must not become discouraged. Check for improvements daily to encourage yourself. In a younger person, within a week's time after starting on the transition diet, a definite improvement will be noted: the skin is clearer, the eyes are brighter, a general feeling of lightness develops, and the desire for more activity increases. There is a definite psychological lift in all this. One is constantly looking forward to improvements in one's health. The all-absorbing fear of being struck down by numberless degenerative diseases is gradually erased from the mind.

Controlling Weight Loss

Don't be alarmed because you lose weight. "Weight is disease" and all of the old diseased substances must go. However, you should not lose weight too rapidly. If you do, add a baked potato or some melba toast to your meals for a while. Cottage cheese will also help check too rapid a weight loss.

You should continue with the transition diet until a feeling of well-being is established. This can only take place after the greater part of the waste encumbrances are eliminated. The length of time required to attain complete healing will depend on your age and physical condition. When you consider that your present state is the result of a whole lifetime of wrong eating, you should not begrudge a few years spent in healing yourself.

Most people are ingenious with foods, and the menus in the transition diet will not present a problem, for they can be changed to suit one's own tastes. The most important thing to remember when preparing a menu is simplicity. Seasoning foods is not necessary. Learn to bring out the natural flavors of foods by baking or braising in a small amount of water and either pure olive oil or another good vegetable oil. We are extremely fortunate in being supplied with delicious fresh-frozen foods all year around. Salad lettuce is available even during the winter months in most parts of the country, and fresh cabbage, carrots, and celery make a delicious combination. Many salad variations can be built on just these few vegetables. Try shredding carrots and adding freshly cooked or canned young peas, making a dressing with the cooked vegetable juice or a mixture of honey and lemon juice. Experience will show you many other similar combinations.

You should not try the complete fruit fast until you are quite certain that all of the dangerous waste matter has been eliminated from your body. Fruit is a relentless eliminator of diseased substances. Many of us could not possibly undergo this severe type of housecleaning because of our physical condition. Vegetables, both naturally raw and cooked, work thoroughly but much more slowly and gently. The fruit diet in itself is the "proof of the pudding." If you are able to live on it comfortably, without any untoward reactions, you are healed. This reminds me of the case of a middle-aged man who really tried to prepare himself over a period of 3 or 4 years for an exclusive fruit diet. Unfortunately, the "cleansing" was not complete, for the sinuses still contained mucus that had not been completely emptied for years. Apparently, there was also some pus in his system clamoring for release. His experience was very unpleasant because he became poisoned by his own dross. He could have avoided this had he made certain that his system was free of the old and poisonous substances. You can make certain by observing the reaction to a fruit fast of no more than 24-hours duration. If the result is a severe headache, dizziness, bad breath, thickly coated tongue, increased mucus discharge from throat and nose, it is quite certain that you are not ready for a pure fruit diet.

Our tongue is the "magic mirror" in which, as Ehret teaches, we can watch for symptoms during the fast. It is a definite indication of the true condition of the tissues, as well as the internal organs of the abdominal cavity. When the internal organs are completely healthy, the tongue takes on a permanent healthy pink color. Observe the tongues of animals; they are always the same healthy pink. The breath should be absolutely pure and inoffensive. There should be no acid or pus condition. All this is plainly revealed in the "magic mirror."

During the process of elimination, the skin becomes loose and even wrinkled, but this is a natural result in everyone, regardless of age, during the healing crises. The natural foods now being consumed, perhaps for the first time during the person's life, start working to improve and rebuild. Nature wisely takes advantage of this situation and begins "housecleaning." Then, after the sticky mucus is thoroughly eliminated and a clean, rebuilt bloodstream is present, the tissues will regain their elasticity. New and healthy cells of the tissues will fill with oxygen and puff themselves up proudly

111

like tiny feather pillows. The daily improvement will be so obvious that you will surely be thrilled to see it. The texture of your skin will completely change and your body will take on a youthfulness that will surprise you. Your muscles will become firm and resilient, and the joy of being alive will fill you with a desire to give your message to the whole world.

Patience and Persistence

It is much better to take your time about this business of healing. It is the most important step you can take in this life. The results are surely worthwhile and all you need do is use some common sense *and follow Nature's rules*. If you start on the road to health the Ehret way, persist until the complete healing. It will provide the essential moral support as nothing else possibly can. Whatever you do, DON'T give up too soon, for you may well be almost within sight of success. As we travel the road of Ehretism, we are not only helping ourselves, but we are also instrumental, through our example, in establishing a new way of life for hundreds of others.

- FINIS -

List of Other Publications

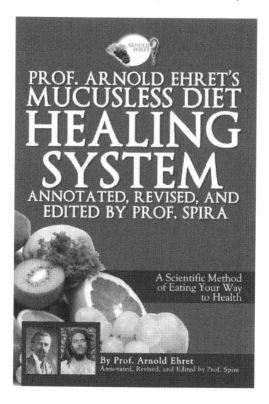

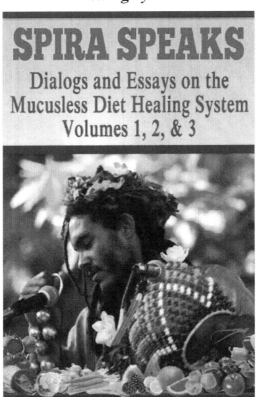

Join Prof. Spira for an unprecedented look into the healing power of a mucus-free lifestyle! After losing 110 pounds and overcoming numerous physical ailments, Spira learned that he had a gift for articulating the principles of the diet through writing and music. As he began to interact with health-seekers on the internet in 2005, he realized that written dialogs about the diet could benefit far more than just its intended readers. This book is a compilation of the best writings by Professor Spira on the subject.

What is the *Mucusless Diet Healing System*? How has it helped numerous people overcome illnesses thought to be permanent? What does it take to practice a mucus-free lifestyle in the twenty-first century? Why is the transition diet one of the most misunderstood

114

aspects of the mucusless diet? Spira answers these questions and much more in his unprecedented new eBook that contains never-before released writings about the mucusless diet.

Visit www.mucusfreelife.com/spira-speaks

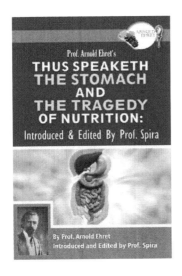
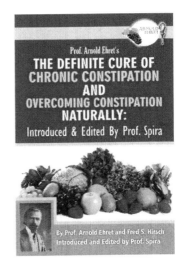

Thus Speaketh the Stomach and A Tragedy of Nutrition

If your intestines could talk, what would they say? What if you could understand health through the perspective of your stomach? In this unprecedented work, Arnold Ehret gives voice to the stomach and reveals the foundation of human illness.

The Definite Cure of Chronic Constipation and Overcoming Constipation Naturally: Introduction by Prof. Spira

In the Definite Cure of Chronic Constipation and Overcoming Constipation Naturally, Prof. Arnold Ehret and his number-one student Fred Hirsch explore generally constipated condition of the human organism.

The Art of Transition: Spira's *Mucusless Diet Healing System* Menu and Recipe Guide

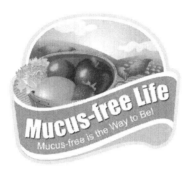

What does a mucusless diet practitioner actually eat? What kind of transitional mucus-forming foods are best? What are the most effective menu combinations to achieve long-lasting success with the mucusless diet? What are the best transitional cooked and raw menus? What foods and combinations should be avoided at all costs? How can you prepare satisfying mucusless and mucus-lean meals for your family?

These questions and much more will be addressed in Prof. Spira's long-awaited mucusless diet menu and recipe eBook! Stay tuned!

Introduction

Purpose

Popular Fruits, Vegetables, and Vegan Items Omitted from this Book

Organic vs. Non-organic

    Mucus-lean

    Raw vs. Cooked

    Satisfying Nut and Dried Fruit Combinations

The Onion Sauté

Filling Steamed and Baked Vegetable Meals

Spira's Special "Meat-Away" Meal

Mucusless

Raw Combination Salads

Raw Dressings

Favorite Mono-fruit Meals

Favorite Dried Fruits

Favorite Fruit Combinations

Vegetable Juices

Fruit Smoothies and Sauces

Fresh Fruit Juices

Sample Combinations and Weekly Menus

Projected Release: Winter 2014

SPIRA'S MUCUSLESS DIET
COACHING & CONSULTATIONS

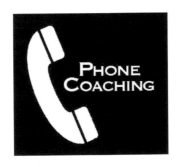

After receiving a consultation with Professor Spira, I was able to take my practice of the Mucusless Diet Healing System to a new level. Speaking face to face with an advanced practitioner was key and a true blessing on my journey. I'm looking forward to following up with another in the future!

-Brian Stern, Certified Bikram Yoga Instructor and Musician

You truly are amazing. You have done nothing but given all you can to help me and I truly appreciate this. Thank you for "feeding me."

-Samantha Claire, Pianist and Educator

"Spira has experienced cleansing on a higher level and passes those experiences to us. He teaches us by EXAMPLE and not only by WORDS, which is rare to find in the world we live in."

-Geargia Barretto, Brazilian Jazz Musician

"When I first contacted Professor Spira for help in practicing the Mucusless Diet, I had many addictions as well as obstructions in my system. I knew it would not be an easy road for me to get started, and I needed help. Professor Spira was able to give me the techniques I needed to start getting out uneliminated feces, black sludge, worms, and mucoid plaquing from my colon and intestines. Within a year

I was completely stabilized and elated to be a lifetime practitioner of the mucusless diet healing system. I felt that good! I also had gained the ability to take this system seriously. He then was able to further guide me in dealing with mental and emotional disturbances, social problems and holidays, as well as work and school issues.

His guidance was critical in helping me navigate a world of mucus, pus, and addictions. It has been almost three years now, and I have the vision and ability to practice steadfastly now, and I have much more work to do."

-Tony Bahlibi, Mucusless Diet Practitioner and Educator

Spira has practiced the mucusless diet and studied the natural hygienic/back-to-nature movements for the past 10 years. During that time, he has advised and helped many in the art of transitioning away from mucus-forming foods. For a limited time, talk with Prof. Spira about your individual needs, challenges, and questions. Skype, telephone, or in-person consultations available! For more information, visit:

www.mucusfreelife.com/diet-coaching

Visit the MUCUSFREELIFE.COM Amazon store for great deals on

Arnold Ehret's Classic Writings

WEB LINKS

Websites

mucusfreelife.com

breathairmusic.com

Facebook

Prof. Spira Fan Page: www.facebook.com/ProfessorSpira

Arnold Ehret Fan Page: www.facebook.com/arnoldehret.us

Arnold Ehret Support Group: www.facebook.com/groups/arnoldehret/

YouTube

Prof. Spira's Breathair-Vision: www.youtube.com/user/professorspira

Twitter

@profspira

@ArnoldEhret1

Visit our Bookstore to Find Books by Arnold Ehret!

www.mucusfreelife.com/storefront/

Spira is now available for mucusless diet consultations/coaching!

www.mucusfreelife.com/storefront/product/mucusless-diet-coaching/

Please Share Your Reviews!

Share your reviews and comments about this book and your experiences with the mucusless diet on Amazon and mucusfreelife.com. Prof. Spira would love to hear how the text has helped you.

PEACE, LOVE, AND BREATH!

36206851R00075

Made in the USA
San Bernardino, CA
15 July 2016